THE AMERICAN ASSOCIATION OF
ORIENTAL MEDICINE'S

Complete Guide to
Chinese Herbal Medicine

THE AMERICAN ASSOCIATION OF
ORIENTAL MEDICINE'S

Complete Guide to
Chinese Herbal Medicine

*How to Treat Illness and Maintain Wellness
with Chinese Herbs*

DAVID MOLONY

Executive Director,
The American Association of Oriental Medicine,
AND MING MING PAN MOLONY, O.M.D.
WITH NANCY BURKE

Illustrations by Michael Brown and Cassio Lynm
Chinese calligraphy by Hui Xiang Pan

Produced by The Philip Lief Group, Inc.

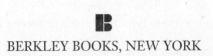

BERKLEY BOOKS, NEW YORK

The herbs pictured on the cover are peonies and chrysanthemums.

This book is an original publication of The Berkley Publishing Group.

THE AMERICAN ASSOCIATION OF ORIENTAL MEDICINE'S
COMPLETE GUIDE TO CHINESE HERBAL MEDICINE

A Berkley Book / published by arrangement with
The Philip Lief Group, Inc.

PRINTING HISTORY
Berkley trade paperback edition / March 1998

The Penguin Putnam Inc. World Wide Web site address is
http://www.penguinputnam.com

ISBN: 0-425-15705-9

Contents

Acknowledgments

The writing of this book, like all the paths that we tread in life, has been a learning experience for me. It started out as a basic nuts-and-bolts guide to Oriental herbal medicine aimed at enabling Americans to use herbs at home for common ailments, just as the Chinese have been doing in their own homes for thousands of years. But the actual task turned out to be less simple than originally envisioned, and while the book remains a thorough primer on the use of herbs, it has become a comprehensive introduction to the ancient and complex theories and philosophies underlying Oriental Medicine as well.

I want to thank my book producer, Judy Linden, for her patience in guiding me from my original attitude—"I have been doing this for sixteen years, and it's really very simple to understand"—and inspiring me to undertake a book that allows people with no background in Oriental Medicine to understand its basic precepts and to use herbs safely.

I also want to thank Nancy Burke, who did an admirable job of absorbing the vast quantities of alien information I threw at her, and setting it all out in a way that makes sense to a culture that is at least ninety degrees off-center from the original. This is no small feat, and I owe the book's ease of use directly to her. Nancy essentially made this book come to life, and if you have read it all, and it makes sense, she is to get credit.

Lastly, I want to thank my incredibly patient and knowledgeable wife, Dr. Ming Ming Pan Molony, who reviewed every word of the book with me, in terms both of its structure and of the clarity and integrity of its writing.

Sometimes I am but a bamboo stalk guided by the winds that are a part of my world.

I hope you enjoy the book and find it useful in your journey to good health.

THE AMERICAN ASSOCIATION OF
ORIENTAL MEDICINE'S

Complete Guide to
Chinese Herbal Medicine

Introduction

Chinese herbal medicine is the oldest and most comprehensive form of internal medicine, and is one of the main treatment components of Oriental Medicine (OM), or Traditional Chinese Medicine (TCM), as it is also called. Herbal medicine has been practiced in China for more than four thousand years, and some of the earliest written documents recovered in that country are about herbs and their use in treating a variety of illnesses and medical conditions. Indeed, some say that one of the chief reasons for the development of written language was to record medical information for future generations.

Both Chinese myth and actual history support this notion. The most important and earliest existing work on Chinese herbal medicine—the *Huang Ti Nei Ching (The Yellow Emperor's Classic of Internal Medicine)*—is believed to have been originally "written" almost five thousand years ago—though the earliest *documented* written records of this work date back to around 200 B.C. Stories and legends about the origins of Chinese herbal medicine go as far back as 2800 B.C.—when herbal lore and practice were oral traditions—to the reigns of the emperors Sheng Nung and, later, Huang Ti.

In those days, information about herbal healing was spread by court physicians whose lives depended upon keeping the emperor healthy.

When the emperor became ill, his doctors tested different herbs and herb formulas on commoners displaying similar symptoms. If a treatment proved to be effective, it was administered to the emperor; the formula was also recorded and shared with other physicians, who would then go on to treat other patients with the same herbs. Although this method of testing was unfortunate for those commoners given what turned out to be an inappropriate formula, the outcome is that we now have a written record of the results of thousands of years of observation and experimentation that is unequaled in the history of any field of medicine.

Since then, over the last two thousand years, the use of healing herbs in China and the system of Chinese herbal medicine itself have been documented and refined in a myriad of important written works. More important, the effectiveness of Chinese herbal medicine has been proven in actual practice on millions of people. In modern China, many Oriental Medicine hospitals contain a panoply of conventional diagnostic medical tools; conversely, an equal number of hospitals practicing conventional medicine have an herbal pharmacy department. Leading medical universities throughout the country have departments in both traditional herbal medicine and conventional pharmacology.

Increasingly, conventional medicine has acknowledged its debt to Chinese herbal medicine, noting that the effectiveness of many modern pharmaceuticals was originally demonstrated in Chinese herbal practice. The wealth of information handed down from Chinese royalty, court physicians, and simple village practitioners about the healing properties of plants and other natural substances is one of China's greatest gifts to civilization.

I first encountered Chinese herbal medicine at the California School of Herbal Studies in 1981 when I was taking an advanced course in Western herbal training. In many ways, Western herbology views a patient's symptoms singly, or in isolation from the functioning of the rest of his body. Diagnosis is categorical. Treatment consists of using single herbs. It is swift and expedient—disease or illness is the "bad guy," and has to be "killed." The philosophy of Western herbology often parallels that of conventional medicine in this way.

Chinese herbal medicine takes an entirely different approach. The patient is rarely viewed simply as his illness or as a collection of isolated symptoms. Rather, he is viewed as a "whole" and intricate system of complementary properties—positive and negative. Similarly, the healing herbs used in traditional Oriental Medicine have a specific, innate property associated with them—described here as the herb's "nature." An herb's "nature" may be more *yin* (cooling, moistening) or more *yang* (warming, drying). In Oriental herbal medicine, herbs are often combined into formulas, and the characterization of the "nature" of the herbs provides insight into how to use and combine them properly.

In optimal health, the complementary properties in the body work together in equally important and sometimes subtle ways to keep the total life energy—or Qi—of the body in balance. Disease or illness, then, is taken as a cue that the body's balance has been disturbed for some time. Thus a person experiencing an "imbalance" may be characterized, for example, as having excessive yang or deficient yin. Specific yin or yang imbalances—or ailments—diagnosed by an Oriental Medicine practitioner are then treated with specific Chinese herb formulas—either more yin or yang in nature—to counteract the imbalance. The aim is to bring the whole body back to a balanced state, allowing it to heal itself naturally and more rapidly.

During my studies, I found myself increasingly drawn to the principles of Chinese herbology, and I immersed myself in all of Oriental Medicine's diverse styles of treatment: acupuncture, herbs, bodywork, diet, and lifestyle counseling. This multidisciplinary approach increased my understanding of how the various components of Oriental Medicine interrelate. That, in turn, led me, as an Oriental Medicine practitioner, to develop faster, safer, and more effective ways of helping people learn to heal themselves, and to bring themselves into balance, or health.

The American Association of Oriental Medicine (AAOM) is a nonprofit organization of Oriental Medicine practitioners dedicated to the premise that rather than simply "removing" disease, it is far better to treat the whole person, teaching them how to achieve an overall more balanced physical state. Therein lies true health and happiness.

The path to optimal health and well-being can be a fascinating and ultimately rewarding journey. This book, the fruits of my fifteen years of experience as a Chinese herbal medicine practitioner, represents the first step of that continuing journey.

Here you will find the basic ideas and theories behind Chinese herbal medicine, including a history of Chinese herbology, and a new look at the old tradition through the eyes of modern science. We will explore the fundamental precepts of Chinese energy medicine, including the concepts of Qi, yin and yang, and hot and cold imbalances. From there we will move to an explanation of how to diagnose common illnesses—or imbalances—from the Oriental Medicine perspective, and how to treat those imbalances with Chinese herbs in both single and combined formulations, with appropriate dosage and duration guidelines.

Detailed information about over 130 single herbs will be presented, including Pinyin Mandarin (romanized Chinese) names and ideograms, Latin and common English names, full descriptions of the specific health conditions and/or organs affected by the herb (called the herb's "function"), and the best methods of administration. Over fifty combination herbal formula preparations will also be presented, with their Chinese and common English names, primary functions, and methods of administration, together with a listing of the names and quantities of single-herb ingredients needed to prepare the formula.

Finally, you will find two listings of illnesses and conditions that may be treated with the herbs and herb formulas presented earlier in the book. The first is an alphabetic listing of common, everyday ailments such as acne, headaches, indigestion, and menstrual pain. The second listing looks at less common, systemic health problems grouped under such broader categories as Respiratory Disorders, Cardiovascular Disorders, and Nervous Disorders.

The appendices at the end of the book will point you to reputable herb suppliers throughout the United States and to further reading materials in the field. A glossary of common terms used in Oriental Medicine is also provided.

The AAOM Home Guide to Chinese Herbal Medicine will give you both a thorough understanding of the basics of Oriental Medicine and the tools with which to begin the challenging journey of self-healing through Chinese herbs—either alone or in consultation with your Oriental Medicine practitioner. More important, it will open your eyes to a new way of looking at health, wellness, and living a balanced life.

May your journey be filled with health, happiness, and balance.

DAVID MOLONY

CHAPTER ONE

Oriental Herbal Medicine: Yesterday, Today, and Tomorrow

The Move Toward Natural Health Care

It is only in the last fifteen years or so that mainstream Westerners have begun discovering and using the diverse healing methods that Oriental Medicine has to offer. Such treatment methods as acupuncture and therapeutic massage—long popular in the U.S. among alternative health-care practitioners—are increasingly used in conventional medical settings, and are sometimes even reimbursed by insurance companies. More nurses are being trained every year in "therapeutic touch," an Oriental massage technique that relieves pains and hastens recovery. Classes in Eastern meditation techniques and t'ai chi chuan are regularly offered at HMOs, local YMCAs, and neighborhood guilds—and they are filled to capacity with an astonishing variety of people: young teens hoping to improve athletic performance, octogenarians keeping flexible and fit, burned-out CEOs trying to ward off a first heart attack, and spiritual seekers of every denomination exploring the power of meditation.

What the gentler, more natural, yet remarkably effective healing methods of Oriental Medicine have in common is this: They put the *individual* in control of his or her own health, *not* the physician. That was a revolutionary concept fifteen years ago, and it still is today.

Moreover, all the healing disciplines of Oriental Medicine promote the idea that ultimate wellness results equally from a healthy body, a healthy mind, and a healthy spirit. That, too, was, and is, a revolutionary concept, and it's a comforting one, too. Rarely is anyone "sick" in all three areas, and increasingly, people who are faced with the challenge of physical illness, and the rigors of some conventional medical treatments, turn to alternative healing methods as adjunctive therapies. People who learn how to to harness the inherent healing potential of their minds and spirits through disciplines like prayer, meditation, gentle exercise, and relaxation techniques can better manage pain, enhance their physical recovery, and sometimes even effect a cure.

Perhaps it is no coincidence, then, that as Oriental Medicine has become more available and attractive to Westerners, interest in all holistic types of health care together with a demand for more natural, less invasive forms of treatment has grown as well. In particular, people have been wanting safer and more natural drugs. They are less inclined to reach reflexively for the latest pharmaceutical panacea. Unquestionably, many pharmaceutical drugs save lives, and many other drugs make living easier. But most drugs only help for the short term, in a very limited fashion, and they often cause new, disturbing, complex, and potentially catastrophic problems. The acetaminophen tablets people take every day for chronic headaches may also, when combined with enough alcohol, cause liver failure. Aspirin may decrease the chance of blood clotting, but they aggravate the stomach and may cause excessive bleeding when an accident occurs or surgery is needed. Heart medications like calcium channel blockers and beta-blockers lower blood pressure and keep arteries from spasming, but they can also cause water retention, fatigue, dizziness, weight gain, and impotence. And many drugs need to be taken for life. The trade-offs in conventional drug care, therefore, can be staggering. Moreover, prescription and over-the-counter drugs grow prohibitively more expensive every year.

There is another route to good health, a complementary, alternative approach to conventional drug treatment that is safer, gentler, more natural, and less invasive. Treatment is relatively short-term and remarkably effective. Moreover, this alternative approach has stood the test of time for over four thousand years.

That safer and gentler route to good health and well-being is Oriental herbal medicine, a preventive and curative form of natural health care that has proven its effectiveness among millions of people through five millennia. The following brief history should demonstrate why

Oriental herbal medicine has taken its place as one of our most powerful tools for good health and balanced living.

Oriental Medicine in Antiquity

The roots of Chinese herbal medicine are long and deep, stretching back to a time before recorded history, a time of myth and fanciful folklore that is shrouded in equal parts legend, conjecture, and fact. It was a time when reclusive holy men living in isolated mountain hermitages began to search among wild plants and flowers for a magical elixir that would bestow eternal life. Although they never did find this "golden bullet" that would endow them with immortality (as far as we know!), their experiments with plants and flowers yielded a far greater legacy. These obscure and nameless monks and hermits discovered that many plants and flowers had powerful preventive, healing, and strengthening properties. It wasn't long before they came down from their mountaintops and shared their newfound knowledge with local villagers and village medicine men.

The news of herbal medicine's immense powers soon spread from villlage to village as tribes traded with each other and met to celebrate various rituals. In fact, on the carved bones and shells found in digs from as far back as 1500 B.C., archeologists have discovered etchings that refer to herbs and illnesses—ancient prescriptions as it were. Officially written historical and scientific records, however, did not appear until almost 200 B.C.

Herbal medicine's origins are usually credited to two legendary Chinese emperors, Sheng Nung and Huang Ti. Although most scholars believe that these rulers and the stories that surround them are largely mythical, much of the extraordinary and seminal work in herbal medicine that was credited to them has been validated by archaeological evidence.

The Divine Plowman

Emperor Sheng Nung, whom the Chinese honor as the father of agriculture and fondly remember as the "Divine Plowman," began his reign in about 2800 B.C. He also is believed to be the source of what would become China's great yin-yang principle—the fundamental doctrine of two opposing but equal life-forming energies that underlies all Chinese philosophy, art, and science. It is said that when Sheng Nung was in the

陰 陽

The Chinese ideograms for Yin and Yang

countryside around the palace, gathering plants for his experiments, he noticed that everything in nature was made up of two currents: light and dark, cold and hot, wet and dry, feminine and masculine, and so on. His observations about nature's two "opposing principles" were thought about, debated, and elaborated on for the next two millennia by philosophers, religious men, and tribal shamans.

More crucial for our purposes, Sheng Nung is credited with the discovery and first systematic recording of the healing powers of plants and flowers. Known as China's patron saint of herbology, he is said to have made daily forays into the countryside to gather hundreds of plants and test them for their healing benefits. Testing them on himself, he reportedly survived numerous poisonings. The results of his experiments became the basis for China's first comprehensive book on the healing powers of herbs. *The Herbal Classic of the Divine Plowman (Sheng Nung Ben Cao Chien)*, or *Sheng Nung's Herbal*, as it is more simply called, described over 250 plant herbs by their taste, functions, and health benefits and listed over 150 illnesses that herbs can successfully treat. And while the first *written* record of *The Herbal Classic of the Divine Plowman* did not appear until almost 100 B.C.—the work of an unknown historian—the information attributed to the original *Sheng Nung's Herbal* is nevertheless remarkable in its accuracy.

Sheng Nung described the guiding principle for combining herbal formulas, a principle that remains valid today: every formula must have at least one primary active herb that targets the illness being treated, but it must also have several secondary herbs that enhance the action of the primary herb and/or prevent adverse side effects. Many of his discussions of the actions and effects of specific herbs have been verified in modern labs around the world. For example, he claimed that ginseng—a herb about which whole books have now been written— "strengthened mentality, relaxed stress, and calmed the nerves." Today, no one disputes ginseng's effects on the central nervous and cardiovascular systems. Indeed, the active ingredients in ginseng that are responsible for those effects—panaxosides, also called ginsenosides—have been identified.

For twenty centuries, the remarkable information about herbs contained in *Sheng Nung's Herbal* was passed down by word of mouth, both among the royalty of the emperor's court and among local villagers living in nearby towns. Among the educated, herbal medicine's theories and principles would be tested, refined, and ultimately recorded for posterity. Among the commoners, local practitioners would test herbal medicine's effectiveness over and over again among large numbers of people. Thus the more esoteric work being done among the affluent was substantiated among the common folk.

The Yellow Emperor

The second emperor critical to the origins of Chinese herbal medicine was Huang Ti, the Yellow Emperor, who began his reign in 2687 B.C. Huang Ti is credited with inventing the first wheeled vehicles, ships, money, and the system of musical notation as well. He was also the first of China's emperors to establish a formal royal court, with cabinet members and royal physicians, the latter of whom would have an enormous impact on the evolution of herbal medicine.

Legend has it that it was the Emperor Huang Ti, together with his most trusted court physician, Qi Bo—both inspired by Sheng Nung's pioneering work with herbs—who developed the first detailed, systematic framework for diagnosing many different kinds of illnesses. They then listed the specific herbs useful in treating those illnesses. More than that, they established Oriental Medicine as a complete and holistic medical system. Their extraordinary work became known as the *Huang Ti Nei Chin*, or *Nei Ching* for short, usually translated as *The Yellow Emperor's Classic of Internal Medicine*. It is not only the earliest extant work on the guiding principles of Oriental Medicine, but it is also one of the most important of the ancient Chinese medical texts, and is still regularly consulted today by authors and practitioners.

Written as an imaginary dialogue between Huang Ti and Qi Bo, the *Nei Ching* discusses Oriental Medicine in large theoretical and philosophical terms, first as a general way of life, and second as a system of complete wellness that necessarily impacts on every aspect of an individual's life. The *Nei Ching* also discusses specific healing disciplines within Oriental Medicine that are crucial to good health, among them the use of herbs, diet, and acupuncture. Though it, like *Sheng Nung's*

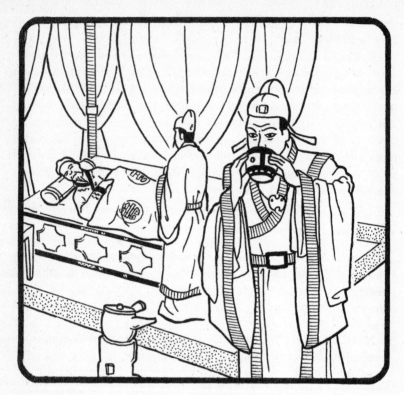

An emperor and his physicians

Herbal, was not formally written down for another two thousand years, its extraordinary store of knowledge became the basis for some of China's most seminal medical texts. The *Nei Ching's* knowledge was preserved orally and passed down through a succession of royal court physicians who left their own indelible marks on the evolution of herbal medicine.

Herbal Medicine in the Ancient Royal Court

Several royal court physicians and scholars are remembered for their contributions to herbal medicine.

Yi Tuen, a royal chef in the court of Emperor Shen Tong Wong (about 1600 B.C.) during the Shang dynasty, is credited with inventing the popular technique of herbal decoction (called *tang* in Chinese and literally meaning "broth"). Decoction is the process of boiling down herbs so that the resultant liquid may be used in soups and tonics. Yi Yuen is said to have shared his knowledge about herbs and decoction, together with many of his personal herbal formulas, with the common people, and modern excavations of a Shang dynasty farm village unearthed more than thirty different kinds of plant seeds commonly used for medicinal purposes, including apricot seeds (*xing ren*), which are used to treat bronchitis and asthma (see page 84). It was also during this period that the words for doctor (*yi*) and for medicine (*yao*) first appeared.

In the Zhou dynasty that began about five hundred years later, a time when formal records about Oriental medicine and philosophy were finally appearing in written form, another court physician, Zhou Li, referred to the "five tastes" of herbs that can be used to heal illnesses. Today, herbs are still primarily classified by their five tastes—sour, bitter, sweet or bland, spicy, and salty (see Chapter Four). Later in the Zhou dynasty, between 600 and 500 B.C., the Chinese term for herbal medicine—*ben cao*—first appeared and continues to be used to this day. (*Ben* means plant with a firm or rigid stalk, while *cao* refers to any grasslike plant.)

Near the end of the great Shang-Zhou dynasties, one of China's greatest ancient physicians, Pin Choi, discovered and promoted the science of *sphygmology*—reading the pulses throughout the body and measuring pulse abnormalities as a way to diagnosis illnesses. Pin Choi wrote several books on the subject, including the nine-volume *Pin Choi Nai Chien*, and in modern times, pulse reading—a complex science *and* art—is one of the fundamental diagnostic tools used by Oriental Medicine practitioners (see Chapter Three). Pin Choi also deserves mention for his work among the common people as well as among the royalty, and for sharing new and updated information about herbs and herbal treatments with village practitioners. Thus, theory and practice were joined in the last years of the Zhou dynasty, and the wealth of information about herbal medicine was substantially augmented and refined. This pivotal time in the evolution of herbal and Oriental medicine presaged the extraordinary developments of the great Han dynasty, when philosophy, spirituality, and medicine merged.

Confucius, Lao-tzu, and The Way

In the years between about 400 B.C. and 200 B.C., all of Oriental Medicine, and herbal medicine with it, underwent a subtle but significant

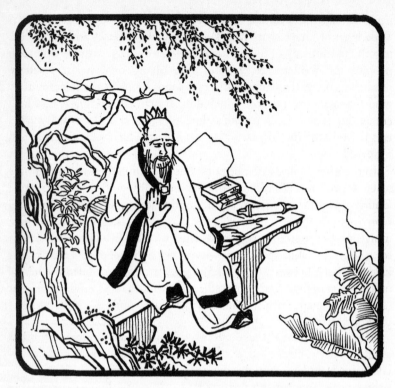

The philosopher Lao-tzu, father of Taoism

metamorphosis. No longer were they *just* about disease and good health. Oriental Medicine merged with a larger and more encompassing Chinese system of philosophy and spirituality that defined all of life, and health as part of life, not simply in physical terms, but as a function of body, mind, and soul working in harmonious tandem.

China's two greatest philosophers, Confucius and Lao-tzu, were instrumental in this movement. They picked up on Sheng Nung's millennia-old theory of nature's two opposing principles, added their own deeply felt and richly poetic beliefs about life, and transformed Sheng Nung's rudimentary treatise into a full-fledged philosophy. Yin and yang were "born," and Confucius and Lao-tzu are credited with synthesizing and popularizing China's unique vision of universal life as an ongoing dance between harmony and disharmony.

Confucius believed that there was an inherent harmony and order to everything in the universe, and this harmony was dependent on the right balance between yin and yang energies. (See Chapter Two for a full description of yin and yang.) Humans play a crucial part in that balance because human actions—good or bad—have an inherent energy of their own. By their good or bad actions, therefore, humans contribute to the delicate interplay of yin and yang, and thus to the ultimate harmony of the universe. From Confucius's basic philosophical beliefs, a complex and far-reaching system of rules of behavior was established to encourage humankind always to strive for the best and most harmonious actions. It followed that good health, like good action, was an essential part of the larger harmony of the universe.

China's other preeminent philosopher, Lao-tzu, the father of China's great spiritual and philosophical system of belief, Taoism, took Confucius's notion of universal harmony and brought it down to a more personal level. Simply put, Lao-tzu said that "as in the universe, so, too, in man." Universal harmony is meaningless without personal harmony. And just as universal harmony and disharmony are manifestations of the perpetual interaction of cosmic yin and yang energy, so, too, is an individual's personal harmony and disharmony a reflection of the ebb and flow of yin and yang energy within him. Man is a universe unto himself. And the Tao, or "Way," as it is literally translated, is the road humankind travels to ultimate harmony inside and outside.

The Taoist principles of universal and personal cause and effect, of universal and personal yin and yang harmony, began to permeate all of Chinese thinking. In Oriental herbal medicine, illness and treatment were now viewed as one part of the great cosmic interplay of opposites and the universal striving toward harmony.

The Han and Jian Dynasties

The Han (206 B.C. to 265 A.D.) and Jian (265 to 560 A.D.) dynasties that followed the era of Confucius and Lao-tzu produced some of China's most renowned and gifted medical scholars. Certainly the early years of the Han dynasty were a golden time in Chinese philosophy, arts, and sciences. A formidable world power that freely traded with other countries, the country experienced long periods of relative peace and stability. In many ways, this period marked herbal medicine's defining monent, when it emerged as a fully formed and all-encompassing medical discipline.

The great physicians and scholars of the Han and Jian eras elaborated on the ideas and information found in earlier works on herbal medicine, but they did so within the new framework of yin and yang, and the Taoist tenets of universal and personal harmony. The works they produced became some of herbal medicine's most critical texts, and many are still mandatory reading today.

The physician Zhang Chong Jin (about 158–168 A.D.), who is known as the Chinese Hippocrates, was the first Oriental Medicine practitioner to categorize illnesses by their yin ("cold") and yang ("hot") symptoms and then recommend the most appropriate herbal formulas to treat them (see Chapter Three). Revered for his work among China's poor, he practiced during the latter part of the Han dynasty, a period of both intense warfare within China and of many deadly epidemics. One of these epidemics was typhoid, a disease that Zhang categorized as a "cold" imbalance. Based on his medical practice, he wrote several books about herbal therapy, the most famous being the *Shang Han Lun (A Treatise on Ailments Attributed to the Cold)*, which is still standard reading today. Zhang made significant contributions to the treatment of typhoid and also developed many well-known herbal formulas, including the classic Rehmannia Eight (see page 213).

A few hundred years later, during the Jian dynasty, the most famous herbalist of the time, Tou Yu Gin (about 452–536 A.D.), a noted Taoist and Buddhist scholar as well as a mathematician, astronomer, and physician, wrote a substantially revised and improved edition of *Sheng Nung's Herbal*. Called the *Ben Cao Chien*, a collection of classic herbal remedies, it describes the characteristics of over seven hundred herbs, including their nature, where they can be found, and how they should be collected.

The Tang Dynasty

Tou's extensive reworking of the classic *Sheng Nung Herbal* was a precursor of the world's first pharmacopoeia, which would be commissioned by the Chinese emperor one hundred years later during the golden age of the Tang dynasty. In 659 A.D., over twenty scholars in the royal court completed the first edition of the *Tan Hsin Hsu Ben Cao* or *Tang's Newly Revised Materia Medica*, yet another ancient text that is still mandatory reading in traditional Oriental medical schools. The fifty-four-volume illustrated book contained descriptions of 850 Chinese herbs and detailed each herb's origin, method of collection, character, taste, effect, and therapeutic use. Revised several times over the next seven hundred years to include over one thousand herbs, *Tang's Materia Medica* not only had a significant influence on Chinese medicine, but it came to the attention of many of China's trading partners and was translated into several languages.

Another great medical figure of this time was the eminent physician/monk, Sun Szu Miao (about 581–682 A.D.). An esteemed and deeply religious Taoist and Buddhist scholar, Sun Szu Miao was revered for his work on treating the illnesses of women and children as well as for his unique insights into herbal medicine, to which he brought the strong Buddhist sensibility of compassion and equal treatment of all individuals. This latter has become a tenet of traditional Oriental Medicine. One of the few physician/scholars who would not work directly under the auspices of the emperor, he lived in seclusion in the Tapo Mountains all his life. Nevertheless, by the time of his death at the age of 101, he had written numerous books on herbal medicine, including the classic *Ts'ien Chin Fang* (*1,000 Precious Recipes*).

The Ming Dynasty

While many seminal works on Oriental and herbal medicine were written after the publication of *Tang's Newly Revised Materia Medica*, the last and perhaps greatest appeared near the end of the Ming dynasty, the work of the renowned physician Li Shih Chen (1518–1593 A.D.). After thirty years of studying nearly every type of plant and other herbal medicine known at the time, and after reading more than eight hundred reference works, Li compiled all his research into a new, fifty-two–volume materia medica that became known as the *Ben Cao Kong Mu* (*Compendium of Materia Medica*).

Li's *Ben Cao* includes almost two thousand medicinal herbs classified into sixteen major groups. Each herb is meticulously detailed according to appearance, "nature," "taste," "hot" and "cold" properties, method of preparation, and therapeutic use. Over a thousand plant herbs are included, as are eight hundred other herbs derived from animal and mineral sources. The extensive appendix includes over eleven thousand formulas classified into four groups according to the number of herbs used within the formula. Many single-herb formulas were also included, together with numerous traditional family formulas that had been passed down from generation to generation.

Li's *Ben Cao* was published in 1596 and brought to Europe in the 1600s, where it was first translated into Latin and later into English, French, and German, among other languages. Today it ranks with both the *Nei Ching* and *Sheng Nung's Herbal* as one of the three most important books about Chinese medicine.

Oriental Medicine: 1644–1911

The three-hundred-year Chin dynasty (1644–1911) that followed the publication of the *Ben Cao* marked the beginning of the great Chinese empire's decline. It was a period that was characterized by tremendous social and political upheavals, foreign influence, and foreign domination. The Manchus, who had invaded from Manchuria in China's most remote northeast corner, conquered and ruled the country for 250 years, but they were never accepted by the common Chinese people, and the country became increasingly fractured by political, religious, and social problems.

In the midst of all this, Oriental Medicine, and herbal medicine in particular, was beginning to suffer the consequences both of royal elitism and social unrest. It now became the exclusive domain of the emperor. Instead of exchanging information with local practitioners, royal physicians now worked solely for the emperor, and within a very narrow framework at that. Relatively little new work in the field was encouraged, and what was produced were mainly antiseptic rehashings of earlier works.

In the meantime, few new doctors or practitioners were being trained to serve the commoners, many of whom were now forced to turn to soothsayers, sorcerers, and even charlatans. Herbal medicine began to take on an aura of "black magic," an association that traditional Oriental Medicine's physicians and scholars had been fighting for centuries. Soon, even the elite of China turned to more occult forms of "medicine" and abandoned the classic way.

The Western Influence

In 1601, Jesuit missionaries from the West arrived in the city of Peking, bringing with them not only their religious convictions and missionary fervor, but a wealth of new information culled from Western science and medicine. However, before they could expose the Chinese people to their new ideas, the reigning emperor, Kang Hsi, suppressed the spread of this new information and made it the exclusive domain of the royal elite. Thus began a significant schism, one that would reach its apex in the early years of the Republic, between the educated upper classes of China, who possessed new and potentially useful information about medicine and science, and the peasant population, who were now completely dependent on local and often untrained practitioners with whom the new information was not shared.

During the Manchus' reign, China was increasingly exposed to the West through its vigorous sea trade and an influx of Western visitors. Newly arrived Protestant missionaries were more successful than the Jesuits in spreading the news about Western medicine, and the gap between the elite and the commoners, between a more Western-based medicine and the traditional way, grew wider. Finally, more and more educated Chinese were traveling to the West and returning home with innovative ideas and information. The pump was primed for the emergence of modern China.

Oriental Medicine: 1900–1949

The Boxers were a secret society within China who attempted, often violently, to rid the country of its Western social and religious influences. The irony of the 1900 Boxer Rebellion was that instead of preserving traditional Chinese culture, it ushered in the age of the New China, in which all things Western, most notably medicine, were embraced. After years of internal social and political upheaval, China's educated elite and middle class, who would later become the mainstays of its Republican forces, wanted to bring back stability, peace, and prosperity. They were less concerned with preserving the old ways than with catching up with the West.

It was during the period of China's Republic (1912–1949) that traditional Oriental herbal medicine, for all intents and purposes, went undergound and was practiced *only* by the peasant population and lower classes. Even if they had been inclined to use Western medicine—and they weren't—it was unavailable to them. Among the upper and middle classes of the Republic, however, herbal medicine had fallen out of favor. Few traditional Oriental Medicine practitioners were being trained, and one traditional medical school after another was shut down, often amid protests by the people. Despite these protests, by 1949, when the Communists took power in China, only eight traditional medical schools still remained open.

Oriental Medicine: 1949 to the Present

Of course, traditional herbal medicine never disappeared completely in China, nor could it. The empirical evidence alone of its effectiveness was overwhelming. Chinese herbal medicine worked, it worked remarkably well, and it often worked when other remedies were either ineffective or unavailable.

The leaders of China's new People's Republic were among the first to publicly reacknowledge herbal medicine's effectiveness. Their officers and medics had used at least one herbal formula, with startling success, to rapidly close wounds and stop bleeding on the battlefield during their many years of fighting both the Japanese and the Republicans. (The herbal formula they used was Yunnan Pai Yao, a Chinese patent formula available from Chinese herbal companies worldwide.) For the new People's Republic of China, herbal medicine had proved itself indispensable at a time when Western medicine was almost impossible to come by and inordinately expensive. After 1949, traditional Oriental Medicine in general and herbal medicine in particular both reassumed a prominent place in Chinese society.

By 1954, the new government had officially recognized Oriental Medicine as a "medical legacy of the motherland." That year, traditionally trained practitioners and Western-trained physicians met together for the first time in Shanghai, under the auspices of the country's Chinese Medical Association, to share their knowledge and to find common ground. It was a momentous occasion for both groups. Traditional practitioners were forced to look at their own discipline in light of newer "scientific" methods, and they began to divest traditional Oriental Medicine of the last vestiges of what was considered "witchcraft." The meeting was equally eye-opening for Western doctors, who were forced to acknowledge the extraordinary effectiveness of many traditional medical treatments, all of which predated their own brand of science by thousands of years.

In the decades that followed, special training hospitals in traditional Oriental Medicine were set up in all major cities across China. Universities of traditional medicine were also established, together with an Academy of Acupuncture and a Central Research Institute of Traditional Medicine. Soon, conventional medical doctors and traditional practitioners were working alongside one another in clinics and hospitals throughout the country. Oriental Medicine was revitalized in the new China and openly encouraged and supported by the new regime, though rulers often imposed their socialist ideologies upon it and obscured its deeper spiritual and philosophical tenets. During this period, many classic Chinese medical texts were finally translated to English and other languages, and their store of astonishing knowledge was spreading to scholars and scientists around the world.

Oriental Medicine Today

In 1972, the remarkable healing powers of traditional Oriental Medicine were brought to the attention of mainstream America in a most dramatic fashion. *New York Times* editor James Reston was part of the press contingent covering then-President Nixon's state trip to China when he had to undergo an emergency appendectomy. Later, he wrote a series of articles about how he had had a painless recovery from the surgery as a result of acupuncture treatment. He also reported on the course of his recovery under the care of traditional Chinese practitioners; it had been far more rapid and pain-free than a comparable stay in a Western hospital would have been. Reston's reports fanned a growing interest in traditional Oriental Medicine in the United States and other Western countries, one that continued growing over the next twenty-five years as several other social and economic trends emerged in the West.

The first of these was an explosion of interest in Asian religions and spiritual systems. As more and more Westerners began exploring Eastern philosophies, they developed a parallel interest in other aspects of Asian culture, Traditional Chinese Medicine in particular, because of its strong emphasis on the whole individual—body, mind, *and* spirit. Second, many traditional Asian medical practitioners and teachers, unhappy with the sometimes restrictive regime in Communist China, left that country to teach and practice in Western countries. New Western practitioners were subsequently trained in traditional Oriental Medicine, and they brought to the ancient discipline a decidedly Western orientation toward its practice.

Finally, conventional Western medicine itself was in the throes of controversy. The often dazzling technological and pharmaceutical advances of the previous twenty-five years no doubt saved lives and improved the quality of life for many. However, technology began to take the place of the more intimate physican-patient relationships of the past. The treatment of illness and disease became cold and antiseptic, more narrow and symptomatic in focus. Further, the new technologies and drugs were extraordinarily expensive and often indiscriminately prescribed, as people demanded faster answers to their medical dilemmas and quick, symptomatic relief. As a result, health-care costs rose alarmingly.

"Managed" Health Care and the Rise of Natural Health Care

The birth of "managed health care" and Health Maintenance Organizations in the late 1970s and early 1980s occurred in part to contain the high costs of late twentieth-century medical care. Now large and for-profit health-care corporations controlled the medical care of millions of people. The neighborhood family practitioner has been virtually eliminated in the process, and patients have "lost" their individuality. While HMOs were ostensibly set up to make the best and most affordable health care available to the greatest number of people, the reverse often happened. Health care—and health insurance—became more restrictive, overtly cost-conscious, and very expensive.

A healthy bottom line was the new goal of health-care managers. Doctors were limited by insurance companies in both the time they could spend with patients and the treatments they could prescribe. Patients were limited in their choice of doctors and treatments. In this fast-food type of patient care, little attention could be paid to *people*.

Finally, HMOs established intensely restrictive drug formularies. These were lists of prescription drugs that HMO executives had decided were the most cost-efficient for the therapy they delivered. Doctors could only prescribe drugs from the formulary list. And if patients wanted their drug costs covered by their insurer, they could only receive drugs listed on the HMO formulary. More expensive, and sometimes more effective drugs in the same class were "excluded" from the formulary. Sadly, the choice of which drugs were placed on formularies often had less to do with patient needs than with corporate competition and profitability—for drug companies and HMOs alike. The wheeling-and-dealing that ensued between pharmaceutical companies and HMOs further marginalized the individual and took health care out of the hands of the one person to whom it most mattered: the patient.

Many HMOs have responded to criticisms that they were dehumanizing patients by emphasizing the importance of preventive medicine and by instituting wellness programs. Patients can now take back some control by helping to keep themselves healthy to begin with (and by saving HMOs a good deal of money and material resources in the process!).

The new emphasis on preventive health care in this country is indeed a welcome turn of events, but it contains an inherent irony. Attention to diet, nutrition, exercise, stress management, and critical lifestyle changes (such as quitting smoking) is saving people's lives and improving their quality of life. The irony is that this has led many people to realize that they can take control of other aspects of their health care by treating many of their own ailments, safely, inexpensively, and naturally, on their own terms.

It is surely no coincidence that traditional Oriental Medicine, which has been teaching all these preventive aspects of health care for thousands of years, is now receiving enormous mainstream attention. More important, Oriental Medicine has another formidable tool for people who want a safer, more natural, and inexpensive way to treat their own illnesses. That tool is herbal medicine. As its use and popularity spreads, even conventional practitioners, who have tended to denigrate it, are now beginning to pay attention.

Modern Research on Ancient Herbs

Research in Western laboratories has confirmed many of the millennia-old claims that traditional Oriental Medicine makes about the effectiveness of herbs.

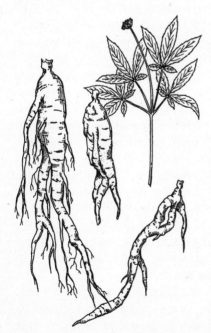

To cite two examples: Gingko biloba (*bai guo*), one of Oriental Medicine's premier herbs (see page 125), recently passed stringent Food and Drug Administration testing for its effectiveness in treating people with Alzheimer's disease. Gingko, long known in traditional medicine for its ability to increase cerebral functioning, had a remarkable and measurable effect in enhancing brain function in Alzheimer's patients, one that was substantiated by MRIs (magnetic resonance imaging) of patients' brains.

Ginseng (*ren shen*), the most famous herb in traditional Oriental Medicine (see page 125), has been the subject of entire books and received perhaps more clin-

Ginseng root and leaf

ical testing worldwide than any other herb. As a general "cure-all," its effectiveness is undisputed. Clinical studies have shown that ginseng strengthens heart muscle and helps prevent heart attacks, regulates blood pressure, stimulates the immune system, inhibits malignant-tumor growth, and increases cerebral function—among other therapeutic properties.

As Western research on herbal medicine's effectiveness continues, and as more people avail themselves of the great healing benefits of herbal medicine, it has become clear to many practitioners and patients alike that traditional medicine and conventional medicine can complement one another in unique ways. Further, the two have much to gain by joining forces in the pursuit of good health. This trend toward cooperative health care has already begun.

Oriental Medicine: The Future

In 1991, Washington's esteemed National Institutes of Health established an Office of Alternative Medicine that began providing clinical validation of many alternative therapy treatments. By 1993, the *New England Journal of Medicine* reported that Americans were visiting alternative practitioners far more than they were visiting conventional physicians. By 1995, Kaiser Permanente, the country's largest HMO, had already been providing acupuncture to its patients for ten years and was now adding massage, meditation, and acupressure to their wellness programs. At the same time, as reported in the March-April 1997 issue of *New Age Journal*, over fifty medical schools across the United States, including those at Harvard and Columbia, had added alternative medicine courses to their curriculum.

In the view of many conventional practitioners, alternative medicine was clearly a viable and important discipline that could no longer be dismissed as a passing fad. Despite the fact that almost 50 percent of conventional medical practioners and insurance providers still actively discouraged their patients and subscribers from seeking alternative treatments, another 50 percent were seeking innovative ways to combine traditional and conventional medicine.

Perhaps the strongest indication that alternative medicine was here to stay was seen just in the last year. As reported in *New Age Journal's* March-April 1997 issue, Oxford Health Plans, one of the U.S.'s most successful and rapidly growing managed health-care providers, with almost one and a half million subscribers in the northeast, announced that it would start offering herbal medicines by mail order. This was in response not only to subscriber demands, over one third of whom were already using some form of alternative medicine, but also to their employees' demands. Further, Oxford had already begun providing their members with other alternative medicines, including acupuncture, Chinese herbal diagnosis and treatment, massage therapy, and yoga.

What does this mean for the future of alternative *and* conventional medicine? In the best of all worlds, alternative and conventional medicine will work hand in hand to offer the finest possible holistic health care to all individuals. Conventional medicine's superlative technological and surgical expertise will most likely remain the standard for treating catastrophic and life-threatening injuries and diseases. Alternative medicine's emphasis on preventive and holistic health, and on safe, natural, and affordable treatments that summon up the remarkable curative powers of the individual's body, mind, and spirit, will help more people to avoid needing emergency treatment in the first place. And when conventional medical intervention is called for, alternative medicine will also be there to hasten and enhance recovery, to revitalize the individual, and to steer him or her toward a new and healthier life.

CHAPTER TWO

Understanding Oriental Medicine: Philosophy of Healing

One of the greatest challenges to understanding and practicing herbal medicine is unraveling the intricate principles that underlie it, principles that proceed from a sensibility that often seems alien to the Western mind. But the rewards of understanding are worth the effort, rendering the task of diagnosing and treating common ailments with herbs easy and natural.

Oriental Medicine As Holistic Medicine

In Oriental Medicine, health and illness are not viewed as static and isolated conditions distinct from other aspects of a person's life. Rather, they are dynamic states unique to an individual and reflective of the whole person—body, mind, and spirit. The Oriental Medicine practitioner is trained to assume that any illness in one part of the body is connected to a vulnerability or weakness in another part.

Basic to this assumption is the belief that people are more than what they seem to be on the surface, more than their obvious symptoms. It follows, then, that in Oriental Medicine, good health is far more than the absence of illness. Instead, good health is a "process," a journey to wellness—and a lifelong one at that—and illnesses are a kind of sign-post thrown up to suggest that perhaps the traveler has stumbled. This deeper and more expansive view of health and illness characterizes holistic medicine at its absolute best. Oriental Medicine always empha-sizes people first—and not just their parts.

Oriental Medicine Versus Conventional Western Medicine

Because Oriental Medicine is essentially holistic in nature, it encom-passes many different healing methods. These methods include medi-tation, proper diet, lifestyle counseling, acupuncture, massage, physicial exercises such as t'ai chi chuan and qigong, and the great body of heal-ing wisdom that is herbal medicine. Each method, however different in approach, aims to integrate body, mind, and spirit as a frontline defense in the prevention of illness, and to celebrate the ultimate wellness that is every individual's natural right.

This multidisciplinary approach to health and illness is in marked contrast to the narrower perspectives and treatment methods of con-ventional Western medicine. In the West, people frequently are seen *only* as their diseases, as a collection of readily categorized and finite symptoms. Cold and clinical dispassion still characterizes too many doctor-patient relationships, and in the conventional physician's mind, people often *become* their diseases. Waiting rooms and examining rooms aren't filled with people; they are filled with "cancer patients" and "heart patients" and "AIDS patients." No wonder many individu-als feel the need to "put on" the symptoms of their illnesses like so many colored armbands that announce their "status" to the world. Even worse, people are encouraged to see themselves as victims of their disease.

Defining patients only by their diseases—let alone labeling them as victims—is dehumanizing and disempowering. And it's bad medicine in the bargain. People who lose their sense of individuality in the face of illness also lose their connection to the vital life force within us all that is so crucial to self-healing. And physicians who ignore the underlying, subtler origins of illness—who cannot look beyond the obvious symp-toms—are also apt to ignore a patient's strengths as well as weaknesses, and both factors are crucial to long-term good health.

Oriental Medicine recognizes that nothing occurs in isolation, least of all good health and illness. The healthy person is not just free of one disease or another. The healthy person is living life at maximum capacity. Like a finely tuned engine, every organic action and reaction within the individual's body is smooth, strong, and unimpeded. All the processes that promote, nourish, and sustain growth and development, and protect the individual from the environment, are operating at optimal warp, and everything is working well together. This fluid and harmonic *balance*, both within and without, is the epitome of good health.

It follows that any illness, great or small, points toward a fundamental imbalance in the individual, resulting in a weakness which allows the illness to take place. The symptoms of illness then become clues to the underlying nature of the imbalance. In fact, the real problem may be far removed from the more obvious ailment.

To use a very familiar example: some people spend their winters fighting off one cold virus after another and never quite feeling well. Treating acute cold symptoms with aspirin, antihistamines, and decongestants may provide quick relief, but unless the underlying condition that leaves certain individuals vulnerable to respiratory infections is treated, "good health" will be only temporary, the cycle of illness will soon begin again, and the side effects of many drugs—even over-the-counter remedies—can create new and more serious problems.

The Oriental Medicine practitioner would view such a pattern of viral infections through a wider lens. He or she would treat the more acute symptoms of a cold—fever and congestion, for example—with cooling herbs, and such short-term treatment would provide rapid relief. But the practitioner would also know that the *initial* symptoms of a cold virus—chills and fatigue, for example—are symptomatic of a deeper condition. This might mean that the individual actually suffers from a more serious imbalance than the simple chest cold would suggest. The goals of long-term treatment, then, would be to eliminate the individual's overall vulnerability to respiratory viruses. One of the ways an Oriental Medicine practitioner might do this is by using a completely different group of warming herbs.

The diagnosis in the above case—that a cold is far more than just a cold—is no felicitous guess. Nor is the choice to use one group of herbs at one stage of treatment and another group of herbs at a later stage. The practitioner's unique approach to diagnosis and treatment is a result of many years of training and a deep understanding of the most basic of Traditional Chinese Medicine's principles: the yin-yang dynamic.

Yin and Yang

Ancient Chinese philosophers, holy men, and medical shamans looked to nature for solutions to the ailments of man. They observed the natural world and saw that everything that has life—humans, animals, plants, the earth, the waters, the atmosphere, the heavens—consists of two mutually dependent and constantly interacting forces of energy. There are the male and female energies of the species; the light and dark energies of our days; the cold and hot energies of our climates; the wet and dry of our atmosphere; the high and low of our earth and seas; the soft and hard, inside and outside, empty and full of the objects around us.

The ancient Chinese called this universal duality the yin and the yang. The yin-yang principle of two distinctive but complementary energies that together create all universal life became the foundation of Chinese philosophy, arts, and science, from antiquity to modern times.

Of all the terms used in Oriental Medicine, Westerners are probably most familiar with "yin" and "yang." Still, the Western understanding of yin and yang is frequently off the mark. In the West, where we are more comfortable dealing with the obvious, the concrete, and the measurable, it is simpler to view the two as separate and distinct energies, one negative and one positive—in effect, the exact opposites of one another. The *taiji*, the universally recognized Chinese pictograph symbolizing the yin-yang concept, seems at first glance to support the Western view:

The symbol for the opposing principles of yin and yang

But the Chinese view is more subtle. From the Eastern viewpoint, the *taiji* says that yin and yang are not so much separate energies as codependent ones. Moreover, yin and yang aren't static—they are fluid, and in constant motion, and the motion is toward each other. There is always some yin in yang, and some yang in yin. Neither exists without the other, and both are essential to the whole.

This concept is even more clearly illustrated in the Chinese ideograms (written characters) for yin and yang. The yin ideogram literally means the "dark side of the mountain." The yang ideogram means the "bright side of the mountain." Yin and yang always have the mountain in common, just to lesser and greater degrees. And in the end, the "bright side" has no meaning without its complementary "dark."

The ancient Chinese assigned to yin and yang specific complementary qualities, or "energies," which were also observed in the natural world. When these complementary energies interact, they form the basic life force or fundamental energy that keeps the world spinning on its axis in harmonic balance.

Yin energy is feminine, cool, passive, and dark. Yin is associated with the cold, the heavy, the moist, and the negative. Winter and rain are yin, and so, too, are the night and the Moon. Yang energy is masculine, warm, active, and bright. Yang is associated with the hot, the light, the dry, and the positive. Summer and fire are yang, as are the day and the Sun.

As in Nature, So in Man

The choice to use images from nature in Oriental Medicine was a conscious one. The Chinese believe that we are microcosms of the larger universe, small worlds complete unto ourselves. Just as yin and yang energies interact in nature—indeed, in all the universe around us—so do they interact within our bodies to provide a primal energy crucial to life, good health, and well-being. When yin and yang work well together, that primal energy is rich, abundant, and apparent to anyone who encounters it. We all know people who are "full of life," or "brimming with energy." We may not be able to measure or even "see" that energy, but it's clear that it exists. We also all know people who seem to have had the "life sucked out of them." We may not understand what precisely has gone wrong with such a person, but we recognize that something is "off balance," that something essential has been lost.

Illness, the first symptoms of which are often marked changes in energy levels, is the most dramatic sign the body gives us that a fundamental imbalance has occurred—either in the body or between the body and the environment. In Oriental Medicine, such imbalances are generally seen as either excesses or deficiencies of yin or yang energy. Various illnesses, therefore, are characterized as excess or deficient yin or yang conditions. Just as illnesses may be more yin or more yang in character, the herbs that treat them are also more yin or more yang in character. In general, yin herbs treat yang conditions, and yang herbs treat yin conditions.

There are examples of yin and yang all around us. To recognize them, we merely need to stretch our minds a bit. Most important, we need to step out and away from results-oriented thinking and look at life as the organic process it really is. We will soon see that the principles of Oriental Medicine are far more familiar to us than we might imagine.

Take the example of a common athletic event like the hundred-yard dash, and view it through the lens of the yin-yang dynamic. Like the earlier illustration of the dark and bright sides of the mountain, everyone in the stadium, spectator and athlete alike, has the race in common—indeed, the race is the thing that holds everyone there. But it is also much more:

> The runners line up at the starting blocks. They bow their heads, still their bodies, gather their energies. The crowd in the stadium is quiet with anticipation. The track ahead is clear. Everyone waits. This passive, cool, receptive state is yin. Then the starter gun goes off. The silence is broken. The athletes leap to the tarmac, a jumble of bodies. Muscles pump, arms swing, lungs expand, hearts beat faster, sweat pours. The crowd begins to scream. This hot swell of motion and noise is yang. Muscles pump harder, hearts beat faster, breath comes quicker, the crowd screams louder. More yang, excess yang. Then the runners break through the tape with one last burst of energy, and the crowd roars. Absolute yang. Gradually the runners slow down. Their heartbeat and respiration begin to return to normal. The crowd settles down, too. Less yang, more yin. The runners stop, they wipe the sweat from their brows and arms, they drink water and pour it over their heads. More yin, less yang. The crowd is quiet. The runners go to their benches, sit, and wait for the next race. The track is clear again. Absolute yin.

And what of that electric feeling of "aliveness" that courses through the stadium? What is the almost palpable but ultimately indefinable hum of energy that moves in and around and through the spectators and athletes, back and forth, up and down through the stands and along the track? That is the vital life force—created by the interaction of yin and yang—that animates all living things. It is what the Chinese call Qi (or chi, pronounced "chee"), and it is the most important of five basic energies in the body that are responsible for good health and well-being.

The Five Energies

The ancient Chinese identified five elemental substances within the body that are critical to the process of physical, mental, and emotional growth, nourishment, and development. They are Jing (essence), Shen

WHEN THE BLOOD IS MORE THAN BLOOD . . .

In this book, as in other works on Oriental Medicine, Blood and the names of Organs are capitalized throughout. This is done, first, to distinguish them from their purely anatomical counterparts in conventional Western medicine, and second, to emphasize the fact that in Oriental Medicine, the Blood and the Organs are endowed with far more functions than in conventional medicine. Indeed, their importance lies in what they *do* within the overall body network, and not in their anatomical structures.

(spirit), Qi, Blood, and the Jin Ye (light/heavy) fluids. For the purposes of this book, we call these basic substances the "five energies," because they are ultimately the products of the great progenitive yin and yang energies. In other books on Oriental Medicine, however, they are sometimes called the body "humors," "essences," or "processes."

The difference in language arises because each of these energies is difficult to define in conventional terms, and in fact, only two of them have a physical character. The other three are pure or "immaterial" energies. Each, however, has a unique role to play in the life of the body.

Jing

Jing energy, also called "essence," is a primordial energy unique to an individual from conception onward. Jing is received from one's parents, and while it has no "material" form, its closest counterpart in conventional medicine would be the genetic material of DNA. Jing governs the slower, developmental growth processes in the body, as well as the rate and degree of deterioration of the body. Strong Jing at birth presages a long and vigorous life. Weak Jing, most often inherited from the parents, frequently manifests itself in the individual as significant immune dysfunctions or chronic patterns of infection. Jing can be strengthened through herbal treatment, diet, acupuncture, and lifestyle changes.

Shen

Shen, also known as "psyche," "mind," or "spirit," is the most difficult of the five body energies to define. It is most similar to conventional Western notions of "soul" or "higher consciousness." Shen is the driving energy behind activities that take place in the mental, spiritual, or creative planes. Moderately weak Shen often manifests itself as anxiety, mild depression, or chronic restlessness. Signficantly weak Shen is implicated in deeper psychological problems, such as clinical depression and psychosis. Shen can be strengthened through herbal treatment, acupuncture, meditation, and physical exercises like t'ai chi chuan and qigong.

Together, Jing, Shen, and Qi are known as the "Three Treasures." When each is strong and all are interacting harmoniously, individuals live life at peak capacity. Everything "clicks"—and body, mind, and soul are fully engaged.

While Jing and Shen don't figure prominently in this discussion of Chinese herbal medicine, a simple understanding of their functions helps us get a sense of the intricate "energy" dynamics of Oriental Medicine. And Jing and Shen are vital considerations in other Oriental healing arts, such as diet, meditation, and qigong. Qi, on the other hand, is the most important of the body's energies, and as such, it is the dominant and recurring theme in *all* Oriental healing arts, most notably herbal medicine.

Qi

In direct contrast to the more esoteric and elusive qualities of Jing and Shen stands Qi—the most dynamic and immediate energy of the body, the "stuff" that animates all of life on a day-to-day basis. Qi is the unique and fundamental energy that results from the interaction of yin and yang. No concept is more critical to understanding Oriental Medicine. It has been called "energy," "vital energy," "primal energy," and the "life force." The Chinese believe that everything in the universe is composed of Qi, from the smallest object we can hold in our hand to the moon that circles our planet.

The body, too, is a wellspring of circulating Qi. Much like an electrical current, Qi energy is in constant and fluid motion: it moves around the body, in and out of the body, up and down within the body. As Qi circulates it transfers its energy to other parts of the body. Thus the Blood, Jin Ye fluids, and eventually the Organs are enriched with Qi. Ultimately, every action and reaction in the body is both jumpstarted by Qi and propelled by Qi.

Qi also has warming properties that are essential to maintaining the body's inner thermostat. And strong, vibrant Qi also has "holding" properties that help keep Organs and tissues in their proper place so they can perform their functions optimally.

On the surface of the body, Qi has a protective role, mediating the potentially ill effects of such external or environmental influences as cold, heat, wind, and damp—Oriental Medicine terms for factors that can affect an individual's resistance to disease (see Chapter Three). Finally, Qi is critical to the process of mixing and metabolizing the food and air we ingest into other vital bodily substances, such as Blood.

These varied and distinctive functions of Qi prompted the ancient Chinese to categorize it in several distinct types, of which the following are some of the most important:

- **Original Qi** *(Yuan Qi)*, also called ancestral or source Qi, is the primordial Qi with which we are born and that is received both from the parents and from the universe.
- **Food Qi** *(Gu Qi)* is received from the foods and liquids we ingest and works with the Spleen to produce Blood.
- **Air Qi** *(Kong Qi)* is received from the air we breathe and is closely associated with the activities of the Lungs.
- **Organ Qi** *(Zheng Qi)* is created by the interaction of Food, Air, and Original Qi. Also called Normal Qi, it is the unique Qi energy that flows through the "meridians" (invisible "channels") on the surface of the body and ultimately circulates through the body's organs. As Organ Qi flows through each Organ, it takes on that Organ's unique energy. Thus, Oriental Medicine uses diagnostic and treatment terms such as "weak Liver Qi," or "tonifies Liver Qi" (meaning to tonify or strengthen the Qi unique to the functions of the Liver). Organ Qi is also essential to the formation of Nutritive Qi and Protective Qi.
- **Nutritive Qi** *(Ying Qi)* helps turn food, air, and water into nourishment for the organs and tissues of the body.
- **Protective Qi** *(Wei Qi)*, also called Surface Qi, circulates on the outside of the body to protect it from exterior or environmental causes of illness or imbalance.

The common imbalances that are manifested as illness in our everyday lives begin as more subtle imbalances in the body's Qi. Identifying these Qi imbalances is one of the first things an Oriental Medicine practitioner does before suggesting an herbal treatment regimen.

Qi Imbalances

Four types of critical Qi imbalances can result in illness. They are:

- **Deficient Qi,** where Qi energy is not strong enough to adequately carry out various bodily functions. (Allergies may be due to deficient or weak Protective Qi. So, too, are many upper respiratory infections, as in the example of the long-suffering cold patient discussed on page 26);
- **Sinking Qi**, a condition of such extreme deficient Qi that a particular Organ no longer adequately functions. (Organ prolapse is a common result of sinking Qi.)
- **Stagnant Qi**, or "stuck" Qi, where the normal flow of Qi either slows down or is actually blocked. (The bruising and swelling of bumps, sprains, and fractures are examples of stagnant Qi.)
- **Rebellious Qi**, a condition that occurs when Qi flows in the wrong direction. (For example, when Stomach Qi flows in the wrong direction, a common result is gastric reflux.)

Blood

After Qi, Blood is the most important of the five energies. In Oriental Medicine, it has greater properties than the circulatory fluid of conventional medicine. Blood is the *physical* manifestation of Qi energy itself. As such, it shares certain of Qi's functions in the body. Most critically, Blood carries nourishment to all the Organs, vessels, tissues, and muscles of the body; it moistens and lubricates the Organs and the vessels in the body; and it enhances mental functioning.

Three basic Blood imbalances can cause illness. These include:

- **Deficient Blood**, a condition that occurs when the Spleen is unable to properly utilize food or Nourishing Qi for good Blood production. (Anemia is a common example of Deficient Blood);
- **Stagnant Blood**, which occurs when the movement of Blood through the body is slow and sluggish. (Pain and tumor formation are frequent results of Stagnant Blood);
- **Heat in the Blood**, a condition which can occur for many reasons, notably internal problems of Yin/Yang imbalance in the body. Blood heat imbalances frequently also occur in tandem with Deficient Blood and inadequate yin. (Constipation is an example of Heat in the Blood).

The Jin Ye Fluids

The Jin Ye fluids are the last of the five basic energies, and like Blood, they have a physical or material property. They also share with Blood similar functions in the body—they are moistening and lubricating— but they perform these functions in very precise ways, beginning with how they are processed in the Spleen.

The foods and liquids we consume are metabolized in the Spleen into two types of fluids, impure and pure. Impure fluids are sent to the intestines for further separation. The pure fluids are sent to the Lungs, and there they are further processed into light or heavy fluids.

The light, watery fluids are called Jin. Jin fluids are circulated by the Lungs to the surface of the body where they work with Protective Qi to moisten the skin and muscles and thereby enhance the defensive role of Protective Qi.

The heavier, thicker fluids circulated by the Lungs are called Ye. Ye fluids are circulated to the Kidneys, where they are separated again into pure and impure Ye fluids. Impure Ye is excreted by the Kidneys as waste. Pure Ye works with the Kidneys and the Spleen to enhance the role of Nourishing Qi in the body.

Two types of Jin Ye fluid imbalances can occur. When the fluids (also called "moisture") are **deficient**, illnesses such as dehydration and constipation may result. When fluids **accumulate**—a condition termed "dampness"—congestion or edema frequently result.

The Meridians

Qi and the other bodily energies and fluids move through the body via an intricate network of pathways that the Chinese call "meridians." These nonphysical "energy" channels run along the surface of the skin and connect the exterior with the interior of the body. Each meridian is also connected to a specific organ in the body. Further, at various spots along the meridians, "invisible" access points provide gateways to specific organs and organ energies. When Qi circulates on the surface of the body, it flows from meridian to meridian, and then from organ to organ, delivering vital Qi energy to every part of the body over a twenty-four-hour cycle.

Of course, trained acupuncturists don't view the meridians or access points as invisible. The body of knowledge that supports the

SYMPTOMS OF DEFICIENCY IN QI, BLOOD, AND FLUIDS

Deficient Qi	Deficient Blood	Deficient Fluids
Tiredness; poor resistance to infections; pale skin; weak muscles; shortness of breath; no or poor appetite; weakness; chilliness.	Irritability; fatigue; poor sleep patterns; easy bruising; pale, dry skin; dry eyes, nails, and hair; dry stools; slow healing; chilly or numb hands and feet; cramps; palpitations; sparse or irregular menstruation.	Dry mouth and throat; excessive thirst; hot flashes; perspiration; night sweats; sparse urination; constipation; insomnia.

SYMPTOMS OF STAGNATION IN QI, BLOOD, AND FLUIDS

Stagnant Qi	Stagnant Blood	Stagnant Fluids
Tenseness; sensation of heaviness or fullness in abdomen, chest, and/or head; pain that comes and goes; indigestion accompanied by belching and flatulence.	Headaches, muscle and abdominal cramps and pain; pain that is constant and stabbing; numbness in hands and feet; anxiety; nodules, masses, and lumps.	Water retention with puffy or swollen face and skin; a sensation of heaviness or fullness in head, abdomen, or extremities; abdominal, joint, and/or muscle pain.

practice of acupuncture is as old as that of herbal medicine—four thousand years—and as meticulously detailed. Both the location of access points (which have a physical correspondence on the skin, where, for example, acupuncture needles are inserted) and the measurable effect that stimulating an access point has on specific organs have been documented for centuries. In fact, some practitioners claim that one *can* see the meridian access points as slight depressions in the surface of the skin.

Many readers are already familiar with the term "meridians" or "meridian points" because of the growing popularity and acceptance in this country of acupuncture treatment. Anecdotal and clinical evidence grows daily, testifying to acupuncture's remarkable effectiveness in treating pain, stress, nicotine and alcohol withdrawal, and many chronic illnesses through the stimulation of specific meridian points with acupuncture needles.

There is a therapeutic relationship between herbs and the meridians, and the energy inherent in herbs and herbal formulas (herbs being essentially yin or yang in character) is connected to the meridian system. In fact, herbs are said to "enter" or have a unique "affinity" for particular meridians. Ingesting the right herbs, therefore, stimulates specific merdians, and thus "treats" their corresponding Organs (just as in acupuncture).

The Organs

The Organs are both the manufacturers and the storehouses of all the body's vital energies, fluids, and biological functions. Oriental Medicine identifies twelve major Organs in the body, each of which has a fundamentally yin or yang nature. Further, each yin Organ is paired with a complementary yang Organ to perform a unique and critical function in the body.

The five yin Organs—the Lungs, Heart, Liver, Kidneys, and Spleen are considered the body's most important ones. They are solid (*Zang*) Organs found deeper in the body and are instrumental in manufacturing, storing, and regulating Jing, Shen, Qi, Blood, and JinYe fluids.

A sixth yin Organ, the Pericardium, is not technically an Organ at all (it is the membrane surrounding the heart), but it plays a crucial role in both protecting the Heart and enhancing many of the Heart's functions. Because Oriental Medicine always places primary importance on process over structure, the Pericardium—like its yang counterpart, the Triple Warmer)—is given Organ status.

The yang Organs—the Large Intestine, Small Intestine, Gallbladder, Bladder, and Stomach—are all mostly gastrointestinal in function. They are hollow (*Fu*) organs found closer to the surface of the body and are involved in receiving, metabolizing, and excreting various bodily fluids and solid wastes.

A sixth yang Organ, called the Triple Warmer, has no anatomical equivalent in conventional medicine. It is more accurately defined as an "energy system" that begins at the tongue and ends at the anus. It is composed of three parts: the "Upper Burner," an area from the tongue to the diaphragm; the "Middle Burner," an area from the diaphragm to the umbilicus (navel); and the "Lower Burner," an area from the umbilicus to the anus.

The Triple Warmer generally enhances the process of ingesting, metabolizing, and eliminating nutrients and wastes, and thus it helps move Qi energies through the body and regulates the function of other Organs. It is also involved in sexual and reproductive processes.

A full discussion of the Chinese Organ system—also called the *Zang Fu* system—is beyond the scope of this book. In Oriental Medicine, entire books have been written on the subject; indeed, there are books on each of the Organs.

A familiarity with the following descriptions of the basic functions of the major yin Organs is all that is needed before we go on to the realm of diagnosis and treatment.

Characteristics and Functions of the Yin Organs

- **Lungs**: Control and regulate vital Qi and respiration; regulate water passage and metabolism; house Original Qi; associated with the skin and hair. (Complementary yang Organ: Large Intestine)
- **Heart**: Controls the Blood and Blood vessels; houses the spirit; associated with the tongue and face. (Complementary yang Organ: Small Intestine)
- **Liver**: Stores and regulates Blood; promotes the flow of Qi; houses the soul; associated with the eyes, muscles, and tendons. (Complementary yang Organ: Gallbladder)
- **Kidneys**: Store Jing (essence) and control reproduction, growth, and development; control marrow, brain, and bone production; control water metabolism; house willpower; associated with the ears, loins, and lower back. (Complementary yang Organ: Bladder)
- **Spleen**: Governs transportation and transformation of Blood and vital fluids; moves Qi; controls muscles; holds Organs in place; houses the mind; associated with the mouth, skin, and limbs. (Complementary yang Organ: Stomach)

This simple but complete introduction to the most basic of Chinese medicine's principles—yin and yang, Qi and Blood, the vital body energies and fluids, and the meridian and Organ systems—should give you the tools you need to understand the methods described in Chapter Three for diagnosing common ailments and choosing the right herbs to treat them.

COMMON SYMPTOMS OF IMBALANCE IN FIVE MAJOR (YIN) ORGANS

Organ	Deficient Qi	Deficient Yin	Deficient Yang	External/Internal Climatic Conditions	Other
Lungs	Weak and shallow respiration, sometimes with shortness of breath; shallow cough; vulnerability to colds; chillness; sweating; sparse white phlegm; weak or soft voice; asthma and allergies; overall weakness.	Fever, sweating, particularly night sweats; dry cough, sometimes with sparse phlegm spotted with blood; flushed or red cheeks; tiredness and weakness; dry mouth, lips, and throat; sensation of warmth in hands, feet, and chest; sleeplessness and restlessness.	Lethargy; poor resistance to colds and flus; asthma, allergies, coughs, and frequent nose and throat infections; tendency to dry skin and shortness of breath.	*Cold-Wind-Deficient Lung:* Aches and chills in head, body, and extremities with no perspiration; scanty clear or white phlegm. *Hot-Wind-Deficient Lung:* Fever with aches and chills in body, head, and extremities; sweating; coughing; thick yellow phlegm. *Dry-Wind-Deficient Lung:* Fever with headache, chills, and sore and/or dry nose and throat; sparse dry phlegm. *Internal Lung Heat:* Pain in chest and ribs with coughing and shortness of breath; thick green phlegm; insomnia and anxiety. *Internal Lung Damp:* Heavy productive cough with large amounts of phlegm and difficulty breathing.	

				Excess Heat (Fire):	Excess Phlegm (Moisture):
Heart	Poor or impaired blood circulation with associated symptoms of irregular pulse and heartbeat; tiredness; shortness of breath; congestive heart failure; pain or labored breathing on physical exertion. *Stagnant Heart Qi*: Nausea, vomiting, difficulty breathing, and sensation of fullness in chest and stomach.	Heart palpitations; pale skin; anxiety; restlessness, and sleep disturbances; dizziness; hot or warm hands and feet; mood swings; night sweats.	Heart palpitations; chest pain; anxiety, restlessness, and sleep disturbances; cold hands and feet; weak and slow heartbeat; sensation of fullness in chest; heart failure. *Stagnant Heart Yang*: Red face; irregular and shallow breathing and pulse; heart palpitations; the crushing and/or squeezing chest pain associated with angina.	Flushed, red face; burning urine, sometimes spotted with blood; anxiety and insomnia; thirst; inflamed mouth, tongue, and/or throat.	Agitation; hyperactivity; mood swings; aggression; blackouts; semiconsciousness; coma.
Liver	Deficient Liver Qi is rare and produces deficient Qi throughout the body. *Stagnant Liver Qi* is common and includes restlessness; pain in chest, breast, ribs, and abdomen; irritability; premenstrual syndrome; depression.	Ringing in the ears; headaches, dizziness, restlessness and numb hands and feet; hot flashes; night sweating; dry mouth, lips, throat, eyes, and nails; red or flushed face and eyes; scanty menstrual periods.	*Rising Liver Fire/Yang*: A severe condition of stagnant Liver Qi characterized by head, eye, and chest pain; dizziness; vertigo; red eyes; nosebleeds; dry stools; irritability; sparse and yellow urine.	*Internal Liver Wind*: A severe condition of Rising Liver Fire characterized by high fevers with convulsions; may lead to stroke, coma, and paralysis. *Internal Liver Cold*: Swollen and/or distended groin and/or testicles. *Internal Liver Hot-Damp*: Little or no appetite; pain or discomfort in shoulders and ribs; fever; chills; jaundice; sparse and dark urine; hepatitis and Gallbladder disease.	*Stagnant Liver Blood*: Irregular menstrual periods with heavy bleeding, clots, and cramps; severe pain, trauma, and masses.

COMMON SYMPTOMS OF IMBALANCE IN FIVE MAJOR (YIN) ORGANS

Organ	Deficient Qi	Deficient Yin	Deficient Yang	External/Internal Climatic Conditions	Other
Kidneys	Incontinence; frequent urination; bedwetting; labored and/or shallow breathing; lower back pain.	Hots hands and feet; dry mouth and throat with thirst; flushed skin; insomnia; night sweats; lower-back pain; ringing in ears; premature ejaculation.	Cold extremities; poor hearing or hearing loss; frequent and profuse urination; incontinence; lower-back pain; impotence.		*Deficient Kidney Essence:* Associated with infertility and poor growth and development.
Spleen	Abdominal swelling, distention, and/or fullness; loose stools; poor appetite; pale skin; fatigue and listlessness; weight gain with fluid retention; menstrual irregularities; varicose veins; tendency to bruise easily. When Blood circulation is affected, there may be internal bleeding, including blood in stools, uterine bleeding, nosebleeds, excessive menstrual bleeding, and hemorrhoids.	Wasting-and-thirsting syndrome of diabetes; severe dehydration with extreme thirst and dry skin, mouth, and throat; chronic and severe weight loss.	Abdominal swelling, distention, and/or fullness; loose stools; excessive urination; poor appetite; pale skin; fatigue and listlessness; edema; craving for hot or warming fluids.	*Cold-Damp-Deficient Spleen:* Tiredness; little or no appetite; diarrhea; lack of thirst. *Hot-Damp-Deficient Spleen:* Fluid retention; thirst; dry, itchy skin; sparse and dark urine; tiredness; little or no appetite; sometimes fever and sensation of swelling or fullness in stomach.	*Sinking Spleen Qi:* Characterized by extreme muscle weakness and breakdown, often leading to prolapse of Organs such as Bladder, rectum, and uterus.

THE ABCS OF ORIENTAL MEDICINE

Vocabulary Recap: To help you remember the terms covered in Chapter Two, here's an at-a-glance glossary.

Air Qi. The Qi received from the air we breathe.

Balance. Good health; the harmonious interaction of yin and yang that produces strong, healthy Qi.

Blood. The physical manifestation of Qi that carries nourishment and moisture to the Organs, tissues, and muscles.

Deficient Blood. Poor or weak Blood (anemia) that doesn't properly nourish Organs, tissues, and muscles.

Deficient Qi. Weak Qi that prevents the Organs, Blood, and fluids of the body from performing their proper functions.

Five Energies. The five basic substances in the body: Jing, Shen, Qi, Blood, and the Jin Ye fluids.

Fluids (Jin Ye). Also called "Moisture." Jin fluids are lighter fluids that moisten the Lungs, skin, and muscles and that work with Protective Qi to help protect the surface of the body. Ye fluids are heavier fluids that work with the Kidneys and Spleen to help Nourishing Qi. Fluids may become "deficient" (e.g., dehydration and constipation), or they may "accumulate" (e.g., congestion and edema).

Food Qi. The Qi received from foods and liquids.

Heart. Yin Organ that controls Blood and Blood vessels. It is associated with the Heart and face. Its complementary yang Organ is the Small Intestine.

Hot Blood. Also called Heat in Blood. Results from problems of yin/yang imbalance control within the body and may be a factor in conditions such as constipation.

Illness. Imbalance between yin and yang energies resulting in further imbalances of Qi, Blood, Jing, Shen, Organs, and/or Fluids.

Imbalance. Illness. Imbalance between yin and yang energies resulting in further imbalances of Qi, Blood, Jing, Shen, Organs, and/or Fluids.

Jing. The primordial energy all individuals are born with, similar to DNA. Also called "Essence." Jing may be strong or weak.

Kidneys. Yin Organ that stores Jing and controls reproduction, growth, and development. It is associated with the ears, loins, and lower back. Its complementary yang Organ is the Bladder.

Liver. Yin Organ that stores and regulates Blood and ensures that Qi flows smoothly. It is associated with the eyes, muscles, and tendons. Its complementary yang Organ is the Gallbladder.

Lungs. Yin Organ that controls and regulates Qi, respiration, and water passage and metabolism. The Lungs are associated with the skin and hair. The Lungs' complementary yang Organ is the Large Intestine.

Meridians. "Invisible" channels that run along the surface of the body and are connected to specific organs. Used in acupuncture as well as herbal medicine.

Moisture. The essential Jin Ye Fluids of the body. (This word is sometimes used instead of "Fluids.")

Nutritive Qi. The Qi energy that provides nourishment to the Organs and tissues of the body.

Organs. The twelve major organs in the body, according to Oriental Medicine. Six are yin organs and six are yang organs. See "Yin Organs" and "Yang Organs."

Organ Qi. The Qi unique to each Organ and Organ function. In illness or imbalance, Organ Qi may be deficient, stagnant, sinking, or rebellious, depending on yin/yang imbalance.

Original Qi. The primordial Qi with which we are born.

Protective Qi. The Qi that circulates on the outside of the body to protect it from illness. Also called Surface Qi.

Qi. The fundamental life force or energy that is found in all living things.

Rebellious Qi. Qi that flows in the wrong direction. (Gastric reflux is an example of rebellious Qi.)

Shen. The "higher consciousness" involved in creative and mental activities. Also called "Spirit." Shen may be strong (calm) or weak (agitated).

Sinking Qi. Extremely weak Qi that can cause Organ prolapse.

Spleen. Yin Organ that governs transportation and transformation of Blood and Fluids and moves Qi. It is associated with the mouth, skin, and limbs. Its complementary yang Organ is the Stomach.

Stagnant Blood. Thick and sluggish Blood that doesn't flow smoothly through the body. (Pain of bumps and bruises are due to Stagnant Blood.)

Stagnant Qi. Qi that is "stuck" and doesn't flow freely.

Triple Warmer. In Oriental Medicine, this Organ is an "energy system" that is crucial to all phases of digestion. It has three parts: Upper Burner (from mouth to diaphragm), Middle Burner (from diaphragm to navel, and Lower Burner (from the navel to rectum). This Organ has no anatomical equivalent in conventional medicine.

Yang. One of the two fundamental energies of the universe. Yang qualities or conditions are hot, dry, excessive, and on the exterior. Yang complements yin.

Yang Organs. The Large Intestine, Small Intestine, Bladder, Gallbladder, Stomach, and Triple Warmer. These hollow (*fu*) Organs are found closer to the surface of the body and are all gastrointestinal in function.

Yin. One of the two fundamental energies of the universe. Yin qualities or conditions are cold, damp, deficient, and in the interior. Yin complements yang.

Yin Organs. The Lungs, Heart, Liver, Kidneys, Spleen, and Pericardium. These solid (*zang*) Organs are considered the most important in Oriental Medicine and are found deep in the body. They manufacture, store, and regulate the body's five basic elements: Jing, Shen, Qi, Blood, and fluids.

CHAPTER THREE

Understanding Oriental Medicine: Diagnosis and Treatment

Before beginning to use herbs and herbal formulas to treat illness, it's important to understand how Oriental Medicine practitioners have joined theory and practice. The first part of this chapter illustrates a typical first visit to a practitioner and the methods he or she may use to diagnose an illness. The second part will show you how to self-diagnose common ailments.

A Visit to the Traditional Practitioner

Your first visit to a traditional practitioner will include a thorough assessment of your physical, mental, and emotional health. In Oriental Medicine, assessment and diagnosis of the patient are complicated processes involving considerable scientific skill and an ability to observe the patient's condition not only objectively but, however much this is possible, subjectively. Symptoms and illnesses are described in several ways related to how yin and yang, Qi, Blood, the Jin Ye fluids, and the Organs are functioning in the body and interacting with each other.

Symptoms and illnesses are primarily categorized in the following ways:

- as essentially yin or yang in nature;
- as conditions associated with yin (cold, internal, damp, deficient);
- as conditions associated with yang (heat, external, dry, excess);
- as imbalances of Qi (deficient, sinking, stagnant, rebellious);
- as imbalances of Blood (deficient, stagnant, heat);
- as imbalances of the Organs (deficient or excess yin/yang or Qi);
- as imbalances of the Jin Ye fluids (deficient or excess)—also referred to as moisture and phlegm;
- as conditions associated with Jing or Essence (weak or deficient);
- as conditions associated with Shen or Spirit (weak or agitated).

Traditional practitioners train for many years in four primary methods of patient assessment: visually observing the patient; listening to and smelling the patient; interviewing the patient; and touching the patient.

Visual Observation

In assessing the patient's overall appearance and physical characteristics, the following areas will be carefully observed:

- **Individual's Body Type and Movement**: Heavier and/or obese people are prone to yang conditions, while very thin and fine-boned people are prone to yin conditions. People who move rapidly, in staccato-like fashion, may suffer from excess heat conditions, whereas people who move slowly and sluggishly may have excess cold conditions.
- **Condition of Hair**: Texture, quantity, and color of hair will be observed. Premature graying, for example, might indicate Blood and Kidney deficiencies.
- **Appearance of Eyes, Lips, and Complexion**: A flushed red complexion with bright eyes and dry lips might indicate a yang condition and possible Heart problems. A pale complexion with drooping, dull eyes and pale or blue lips might indicate a chronic yin deficiency and/or a serious Blood imbalance, such as Blood deficiency, sometimes called anemia.
- **Condition of Skin**: People with dry skin may have a Blood deficiency, while people with edema ("swollen" skin that retains fluids) may be suffering from stagnant Qi.
- **Condition of Tongue**: In Oriental Medicine, different areas of the tongue specifically relate to different organs in the body. For

example, the tip of the tongue is related to the Heart and the Lungs. Observing the conditions of different areas of the tongue provides the practitioner with information about possible problems with related organs and is one of the traditional practitioner's primary diagnostic tools. A pale red or pinkish tongue, for example, is considered normal. A bright red tongue may indicate internal heat problems, a bluish tongue may be a sign of internal cold problems, and a purplish tongue may indicate stagnation. A swollen tongue may indicate a problem of internal damp or a Qi deficiency, while a very thin tongue may indicate an overall deficiency pattern.

Cracks, lines, fissures, and teeth marks on the tongue often indicate problems with related Organs. For example, cracks and fissures near the tip of the tongue may indicate Heart problems. Teeth marks on the sides of the tongue may indicate a Spleen deficiency. (The Spleen "controls" the proper distribution of water throughout the body. When the Spleen is deficient, too much water may be retained and the tongue may swell enough that teeth imprints can be observed on it.)

A thin, white coating (or "fur") on the tongue is normal, but a thick white coating is often a sign of internal cold problems. While a tongue that is pale red (or a "healthy" pink) is generally considered "normal," as explained above, a red tongue *with* a thick or greasy-looking white coating may indicate an internal heat problem. Finally, while a slightly moist tongue is considered normal, a very moist tongue may be an indicator of internal damp conditions. A moist tongue with a very sticky coating usually indicates the presence of internal mucus or phlegm.

When the results of these observations are looked at in total, they give the practitioner a good idea of what the nature of the imbalance is, and whether there is an overall pattern of excess or deficiency.

Listening and Smelling

The practitioner will listen carefully for coughs, wheezes, and congestion. He or she will also listen to how a patient breathes and to the quality of a patient's voice. Rapid breathing and a loud voice may be indications of excessive heat conditions, while shallow breathing and a soft voice may be signs of internal cold.

Some practitioners will also take particular note of a patient's "smells" and the nature of those smells (foul, fishy, or sour, for example) by assessing the patient's breath, body odor, sputum, and urine and feces, either by interviewing the patient or by observation.

Interviewing

The traditional medical practitioner will take an extensive medical history of the patient. Besides obtaining as much information as possible about the patient's current symptoms and previous illnesses, as well as a history of family illnesses, the practitioner will also obtain specific information about a variety of physical, emotional, and lifestyle factors that may not appear related to the patient's specific ailment. These may include questions about the following:

- **Climate and other external causes of disharmony**: The patient may be queried about his or her sensitivity to heat, cold, dampness, and wind, and about related symptoms of fever, chills, perspiration, pain, and dizziness. For example, people who prefer the cold and also experience sweaty palms and soles may have a yin deficiency.
- **Preferences in food and drink**: The patient may also be asked if he or she prefers spicy or bland foods, warm or cold drinks. A craving for spicy foods and warming drinks may indicate an internal cold imbalance or possibly parasites.
- **Digestion, bowel, and Bladder habits**: Both loose bowels and excessive urination are signs of Kidney imbalance.
- **Sleep patterns**: Insomnia may be a sign of deficient Blood and/or a deficient Heart yin, while excessive sleep may be a sign of deficient yang.
- **Disturbances and/or pain in the nose, throat, chest, eyes, ears, and/or head**: Pain and/or congestion in the nose, throat, or chest are related to imbalances of the Heart and Lungs. Blurred vision may indicate a Blood deficiency or Liver imbalance. A high-pitched ringing in the ears may indicate a Kidney imbalance. Chronic headaches may indicate an excessive yang condition.
- **Lifestyle factors**: The patient may be carefully questioned about such factors as smoking, excessive alcohol consumption, drugs (prescribed and recreational), and about social and family relationships as well as work and recreational activities. The physical,

psychological, and emotional effects of these may cause, contribute to, or exacerbate various patterns of disharmony.

- **Sex**: Men may be questioned about sexual drive, impotence, incontinence, and nocturnal emissions. Women may be questioned about sexual drive, menstruation, pregnancies, and gynecological problems.

- **Emotions**: As we discussed earlier, emotions play a crucial role in internal disharmonies. Persistent feelings of anxiety may indicate a Heart imbalance, while chronic anger may indicate a Liver imbalance. A patient's clear self-assessment of his or her overall emotional state is critical to a fuller understanding of her physical state.

Touching

The traditional practitioner "touches" the patient's body in two distinct ways: by palpation and by pulse taking.

In palpation, the skin and various points on the body along the meridian channels are lightly massaged and/or palpated (sometimes with stronger finger-and-hand pressure similar to that of breast examination). Light massage of the skin allows the practitioner to make a general assessment of body/skin temperature and skin moisture or dryness. This examination can confirm a patient's self-assessment of sensitivity to cold or heat. Palpation along the meridian points that correspond to specific internal organs may yield special areas of poor muscular tone, sensitivity, and/or pain that can alert the practitioner to corresponding internal organ disharmonies.

As we mentioned in Chapter One, the science of sphygmology—pulse diagnosis—goes back over two thousand years. It is complex science *and* art that takes years to master. Adept practitioners can detect twelve different wrist pulses (six on each wrist), each of which corresponds to one of the twelve major organs. Further, the skillful practitioner can also distinguish over thirty pulse qualities (weak, strong, floating, choppy) in *each* of the twelve wrist pulses. By analzying these pulse qualities, the practitioner can identify not only current organ disharmonies, but also past imbalances and possible future ones.

As with tongue diagnosis, entire books have been written on the subject of pulse diagnosis. For the purposes of this book, it is important to know that the practitioner will most likely take several wrist pulses (while holding the wrist in various positions) to measure the pulses' depth, speed, strength, quality (choppy or thready, among others), and rhythm (regular or irregular).

After this extensive and comprehensive examination, the practitioner will use the Eight Principles of diagnosis discussed on page 55 to organize symptoms, make an initial primary diagnosis, and prescribe a full course of treatment with appropriate herbal formulas and follow-up visits to monitor recovery and adjust formulas. For long-standing imbalances and more serious, chronic conditions, the practitioner will most likely supplement herbal treatment with one or more additional treatment methods, such as acupuncture and proper diet.

Self-Diagnosis and Treatment: Some Reminders

In Chapter Two we learned that Oriental Medicine views illness as a fundamental imbalance or disharmony between yin and yang energies. We also learned that the interaction of yin and yang energies produces Qi energy, the basic life force of all living things. Yin and yang and Qi energies are constantly interacting, both within the body (affecting Organs, Blood, and other fluids) and in nature (affecting plants, minerals, climate, and other natural phenomena). Everything in the universe, therefore, possesses yin, yang, and Qi energies.

We also learned that different qualities are associated with yin and with yang, among them: cold and hot; wet and dry; external and internal; empty (deficient) and full (excess). We learned, too, that there are different kinds of Qi: protective, rebellious, and nutritive, and so on.

In Oriental herbal medicine, diagnosis and treatment are primarily organized around the qualities of yin, yang, and Qi, and their relationship with the Organs, Blood, and other fluids in the body. Several methods are used. Some, like the Five Elements system, which is used more for acupuncture treatment, are quite complex and require years of training and practice to master. Many of the books in the bibliography contain excellent discussions of the Five Elements and other diagnostic systems.

For this home guide to herbal self-treatment, we use a system that is easier to grasp. First, we identify the causes of imbalance—or illness—from the perspective of Oriental Medicine, and then we use Oriental Medicine's "Eight Principles" to organize symptoms and make a diagnosis. Using the Eight Principles makes an initial diagnosis easier, but it too, takes years of study to master.

The Causes of Illness

In Oriental Medicine theory, almost all illness (or imbalance) is caused either by *internal* conditions, emotional or psychological in origin, or by *external* conditions, "natural" or "climatic" in origin. This book primarily focuses on the physical symptoms of illness that are usually associated with external causes. They are the most familiar to us and the most readily identifiable. They are also the symptoms that most frequently catch our attention and bring us to a practitioner.

It is important to note, however, that Oriental Medicine views the internal causes of disharmony as far more critical than the external ones. Over a prolonged period of time, extremes of any emotion can damage Organs and thus affect Qi and other bodily energies and fluids. This, in turn, can cause serious chronic physical problems as well as make an individual more vulnerable to the external causes of illness. Indeed, a long-standing internal weakness often is the "weak link" in an individual that allows external causes of illness to enter the system.

Internal Causes of Illness

Oriental Medicine practitioners take so-called psychosomatic illnesses seriously. This is largely why Oriental Medicine has always included healing disciplines such as meditation and lifestyle counseling as standard practice. For example, treating the *physical* symptoms of anger—most obviously high blood pressure—is self-defeating if the underlying emotional imbalance is not treated, too.

Further, the Oriental Medicine practitioner is especially concerned about the physical damage that may result from prolonged emotional imbalances. We are, of course, emotional beings. Experiencing a full range of emotions, from the negative to the positive, over the course of our day is natural and healthy. However, when any one emotion is experienced to excess and over a long period of time, the yin-yang balance in the body may be critically disturbed, Qi may become depleted or blocked, and serious illness may occur.

Oriental Medicine identifies seven emotions as the primary internal causes of illness and disease. Each is specifically related to an organ or organs in the body. When experienced excessively and chronically, these emotions can injure those organs and cause corresponding physical illnesses.

- **Anger**: Anger is related to the Liver. Excessive and chronic anger, with all its attendant emotions, such as bitterness and resentment, damages the Liver and may result in rebellious Liver Qi that rises upward. Headaches, high blood pressure, and dizziness may be signs of excessive anger.

- **Sadness and anxiety**: Sadness is related to the Lungs and to their complementary organ, the Large Intestine. Excessive sadness or anxiety damages the Lungs, which, through the mechanism of breathing, circulate Qi throughout the body. Blocked or stagnant Qi may thus result from excessive sadness or grief. Chronic shallow or irregular breathing are signs of excessive sadness, and asthma can be one of the physical results. Where excessive sadness or anxiety affects the Large Intestine, irritable bowel syndrome and other colitislike illnesses may result.

- **Grief**: Grief, the most extreme manifestation of sadness, affects not only the Lungs, but also the Heart (which houses the individual's Spirit), and the Triple Warmer (which regulates all phases of digestive metabolism). Grief can seriously impair the healthy flow of Qi at these organ sites. Frigidity and chronic constipation are sometimes the results of extreme grief.

- **Fear**: Fear is related to the Kidneys, which house the individual's willpower, and to the Bladder, the Kidneys' complementary organ. Excessive fear over time can affect the Kidney's ability to "hold" Qi in place. Involuntary urination—or bed-wetting in children—can be one of the physical results of depleted Kidney Qi.

- **Fright**: Fright, or terror, is an extreme—and usually sudden—manifestation of fear. Fright is related primarily to the Heart, and an extreme physical result of excessive fright might be an acute coronary episode. Acute fright that isn't treated tends to become chronic fear that may damage the Kidneys.

- **Joy**: The excessive "joy" of Oriental Medicine is directly related to the Heart and refers to an overexcited and overstimulated state more closely resembling mania than happiness. Individuals prone to excessive and chronic joy are most often "pleasure seekers" who are overly loud, overly talkative, ceaselessly active, and constantly in search of stimulation. They frequently suffer from overactive Heart syndromes and are subject to heart palpitations and insomnia. In extreme cases, schizophrenia is sometimes a manifestation of excessive joy.

- **Rumination**: Also called overconcentration or pensiveness, rumination is related to the Spleen, which houses the individual's mind. Obsessive-compulsive types who are overly concerned with details and do work that is mostly of a mental nature are particularly prone to the effects of excessive rumination, which can include extreme fatigue, indigestion, acute stomach pain, and obesity.

External Causes of Illness

In Chapters One and Two we described how the principles of Oriental Medicine were derived from observations of nature. All the myriad energy dynamics observed in nature—indeed, in the universe as a whole—were then ascribed to man: individuals became universes unto themselves, subject to all the natural actions and reactions that occurred in the larger world around them. This reliance on natural phenomena to understand illness logically led to the use of a naturalistic language to describe illness. Nowhere is this more apparent than in the six terms used to describe the major external causes of illness.

Each of these terms—sometimes called the "Six Evils" or "Six Excesses," relates to a specific "climatic" or weatherlike condition that is essentially yin or yang in character. The six external causes of illness are: wind, cold, heat, fire, dampness, and dryness. Externally caused illnesses are usually acute, sudden, and confined to or near the surface or exterior of the body. The common cold is an external wind illness whose acute upper respiratory symptoms (runny nose, congestion, scratchy throat, minor aches and pains) are considered surface or exterior conditions.

External conditions may also penentrate to the interior of the body, where they become more serious, chronic illnesses that affect Organs, Blood, and Qi. External imbalances or illnesses, therefore, may have a complementary internal manifestation. For example, an external wind illness such as the common cold may penetrate to the Spleen, causing severe diarrhea and vomiting that in turn may dehydrate the body and cause deficiencies of Blood and fluids.

Further, external causes of illness—and their accompanying symptoms—frequently occur together, and so it is common to have symptoms of both *wind* and *cold* (*wind-cold*) or *damp* and *heat* (*damp-heat*), to use two examples.

- **Wind**: Wind is yang in nature and is related to the spring. Wind symptoms are characterized by their suddenness and their intensity, and include shaking, trembling, unbalanced or jerky movements, dizziness, and joint and muscle pains that move throughout the body.

  The common cold is a typical example of a wind illness—or "injury," as these external imbalances are often called. In spring, when the body's skin is unaccustomed to sudden warmer temperatures and the pores of the skin easily dilate (open), wind is most likely to "invade" the body and cause illness. Indeed, wind's ability to penetrate the body's protective surface Qi makes it the most potent of the six external causes of illness, because it often creates an entryway through which other external influences may enter. Further, the relative strength of the wind injury, combined with any weaknesses in an individual's protective Qi, will determine how deeply an invading illness penetrates the body's interior. And the deeper the penetration of the illness, the more difficult it is to dislodge.

  It is very common for wind illnesses to occur in tandem with one of the other external causes of illness, particularly *cold*. Indeed, *wind-cold* injuries are very common in spring. *External wind* illnesses include the common cold and flu, with coughing, runny nose, sneezing, headaches, dizziness, and muscle and joint pains. *Internal wind* diseases are more serious and are characterized by tremors, seizures, and lack of coordination. Epilepsy and Parkinson's disease are examples of internal wind illnesses.

- **Cold**: Cold is yin in nature and is related to the winter. Cold symptoms include fever and sudden chills, headaches, and body cramps, aches, and pains. Cold illnesses or injuries damage a person's internal yang (or warming) energies and he will usually have a strong aversion to the cold and an inability to get warm. Cold often combines with wind, as noted above. Overconsumption of chilled foods and drinks may also produce cold symptoms.

  External cold illnesses include the colds and influenza associated with winter, but with fever, chills, deep muscle aches and pains, and extreme fatigue. *Internal cold* symptoms may penetrate the body's internal organs, particularly the Lungs, Stomach, and Spleen, causing intestinal or Stomach pain, diarrhea, and vomiting.

- **Heat**: Heat is yang in nature and is related to the summer. Heat symptoms include sweating, dry mouth and throat, water retention, constipation, heart palpitations, inflammation and swelling, and an aversion to the heat and to warm foods and liquids. Red, dry eyes, and rashes, boils, and acne are also heat symptoms. Overconsumption of hot, spicy foods may also produce heat symptoms, as will caffeine and alcohol. Heat often combines with dampness.

External heat illnesses are characterized by constipation, difficult or sparse urination, feverishness, perspiration, sudden skin rashes and eruptions, heart palpitations, and agitation. Heatstroke is an extreme example of an external heat illness. *Internal heat* may invade the stomach, especially in combination with dampness, causing severe abdominal cramping, spasms, and pain, vomiting with a a clammy, chilly feeling, and excessive sweating.

• **Dampness**: Dampness is yin in nature and is related to the late summer. Damp conditions are characterized by feelings of heaviness, lethargy, and the accumulation of dense and sluggish fluid and phlegm. Damp symptoms may include aching, stiff, and swollen joints, a sensation of heaviness in the chest, oily skin, edema, excessive mucus discharge, and abdominal distension and swelling.

External damp illnesses often include swollen and painful joints and edema-like conditions of the skin. Osteoarthritis is an example of an external damp illness. *Internal damp* conditions frequently affect the Spleen and may cause abdominal pain and swelling, vomiting, and diarrhea. Prolonged internal damp can also produce a serious and chronic condition that Oriental Medicine practitioners call phlegm or mucus. Phlegm buildup throughout the body may lead to chronic high blood pressure or neurological problems.

Dampness is mostly frequently seen in combination with external cold, heat, and wind. *Damp-cold* imbalances frequently include poor circulation, stiff and painful joints and muscles, and overall tiredness. *Damp-heat* imbalances often manifest themselves on the surface of the skin as pus-filled sores and abscesses, or the swollen, red, and painful lesions of herpes and shingles. Internal damp-heat is often responsible for bronchitislike conditions. *Damp-wind* imbalances may manifest themselves as intermittent attacks of swollen lymph nodes and hives, or as draining sores and ulcers of the skin. Severe internal damp-wind can impair the function of the brain and circulatory system and may lead to strokes and seizures.

- **Dryness**: Dryness is yang in nature and is related to autumn. Dry conditions are characterized by excessive loss of fluids, dry skin, hair, eyes, lips, and nose, and dry, hacking coughs with little phlegm. Dehydration and constipation with hard, dry stools are common dry imbalances.

   Dryness is especially damaging to the Lungs, and to the balance of Blood and fluids within the body. *External dry* conditions are especially prevalent in hot, dry weather with winds, and may be accompanied by dehydration, dizziness, scanty perspiration and urination as well as injuries to the mucous membranes, particularly the eyes. Hot, spicy foods and many medications, especially allergy medications that are used to dry mucous membrances, can cause or exacerbate dry imbalances. *Internal dry* conditions can seriously injure the balance of Blood and other fluids in the body, leading to an overall systemic weakness, like anemia, or disturbances in sight and hearing.

- **Fire**: Fire is yang in nature and characterizes very extreme conditions of external or internal heat, particularly when they are accompanied by severe emotional excesses, called "inner-fire" symptoms. Inner fire particularly affects the Stomach, Lungs, and Liver. Extreme anger or rage, for example, may "collect" in the Stomach, causing Stomach fire that may rise upward and affect the face, head, and teeth, and in very extreme cases, the brain.

The Eight Principles of Diagnosis

When an Oriental Medicine practitioner does the extensive physical examination and interview we learned about earlier in this chapter, it is not enough just to identify the general type of symptoms or illness a patient is experiencing (heat, wind, or damp, for example). It is also crucial to determine the specific nature of the illness (yin/cold or yang/hot); how far the illness has progressed or "moved" (is it on the outside of the body or has it moved to one of the interior levels?); and how the entire body is responding to the illness (is there an excess or a deficient condition?). Only when all these factors have been considered can the proper herbal formula be given.

   The traditional practitioner categorizes the symptoms of illness in eight principal ways, using yin and yang as the starting point. Illnesses are primarily yin in nature (with internal, cold, and deficient symptoms)

COMMON SYMPTOMS OF EXTERNAL (CLIMATIC) CAUSES OF ILLNESS

Wind	*Cold*	*Heat*
Spasms and cramping with pain that moves around the body; lack of coordination and balance; shaky or trembling hands and feet; shivering; sneezing; itching or painful eyes, ears, nose, and/or throat.	Feeling of coldness in arms, head, and chest, with weakness, paleness, and clammy feeling in face and extremities; aversion to cold; pain in head, chest, and extremities; diarrhea.	Fever and pain with infection or swelling that is often accompanied by a hot or burning sensation; running sores; red or flushed face; red eyes and nose; thirst; discharges; aversion to heat.
External wind ailments include the common colds and flu viruses of spring and autumn.	External cold ailments include winter colds and flus with fever.	External heat ailments include constipation, fevers, sudden rashes, agitation, and heatstroke.
Internal wind ailments include epilepsy and Parkinson's Disease.	Internal cold ailments include above symptoms plus complications of intestinal or abdominal pain, diarrhea, and vomiting.	Internal heat ailments include abdominal cramping with vomiting, clamminess, and excessive sweating.

Dampness	*Dryness*	*Fire*
Dizziness or a feeling of fullness in face and head with thick congestion in eyes, nose, throat, and chest; swollen lymph nodes; labored breathing; nausea; a feeling of fullness in abdomen and chest.	Dehydration; dry skin, hair, eyes, and nose, often with dry and hacking cough; constipation with dry stools; sparse sweating and/or urination; sore eyes, mouth, and nose.	"Fire" conditions are extreme manifestations of any of the other five external causes of illness, but fire is especially associated with extreme conditions of heat, including severe dehydration with fever, skin rashes, red eyes and face, sparse urine, constipation, severe mental agitation, and/or delirium.
External damp ailments include painful joints, edemalike conditions, and osteoarthritis.	External dry ailments include dehydration with scanty urination and sparse or no sweating.	
Internal damp ailments are characterized by profuse phlegm (mucus) throughout body and include high blood pressure and neurological problems.	Internal dry ailments cause serious fluid imbalances throughout body and include anemia and disturbances of vision and hearing.	Internal fire ailments are often caused by extreme emotions, especially anger, and by overindulgence in certain foods and alcohol. Fire especially affects the Lungs, Liver, and Stomach.

COMMON COMBINATIONS OF EXTERNAL (CLIMATIC) CAUSES OF ILLNESS

Wind-cold	*Wind-heat*	*Wind-damp*
Includes external wind symptoms plus additional symptoms of cough; headache; nose congestion; fever; aversion to drafts; joint pains; shortness of breath.	Includes external wind symptoms plus additional symptoms of severe congestion in nose; sore throat; sore and/or inflamed tonsils; red eyes; headache; extreme thirst; anxiety or restlessness.	Includes external wind symptoms plus additional symptoms of aversion to drafts; a sensation of heaviness in head and/or chest; sparse urination; rashes, blisters, and boils; joint pain that moves around the body; sparse urination.

Wind-dry	*Cold-damp*	*Heat-damp*
Includes external wind symptoms plus additional symptoms of constipation, and dry scalp, skin, and nails.	Includes external cold symptoms plus additional symptoms of sparse perspiration and urination; pain and swelling; loose stools.	Includes external heat symptoms plus additional symptoms of fever with sweating, particularly in the afternoon; headache; vomiting; diarrhea; a sensation of fullness and/or tightness in chest; thirst; sparse, dark urine; jaundice; inflammations.

Summer-Heat
Includes symptoms of external heat and damp and commonly occurs in late summer, often after exposure to severe heat. Characterized by sudden onset of high fever and exhaustion.

or yang in nature (with external, hot, and excess symptoms). These are the Eight Principles:

YIN
  Internal
  Cold
  Deficient
YANG
  External
  Hot
  Excess

Yin and yang, as we have learned, are fluid states—there is always some yin in yang, and yang in yin. Symptoms, too, are fluid, and they frequently occur in combination—external-cold, internal-hot, and deficient-yang, for example. To begin to understand how to best match symptoms with the right herbal formulas, a general description of the most common symptoms together with very general traditional treatment approaches associated with the eight diagnostic principles is given below.

In general, yang (warming) herbs are given for yin symptoms, and yin (cooling) herbs are given for yang symptoms. The most frequent exceptions to this rule are the yang-related symptoms of "false heat," which is described last.

Principle	Common Symptoms	Treatment
Yin	Combination of interior, cold, and deficient conditions characterized by paleness, fatigue, weakness, and shortness of breath.	Warm and tonify
Internal	Illnesses affecting deeper tissues and organs of the body, and brain, nerves, and bones.	Dependent on excess/deficiency and hot/cold conditions
Cold	Illnesses characterized by cold extremities, pale skin, low metabolism, frequent and copious urination, diarrhea, and aversion to cold.	Warm and expel cold or pathogen
Deficient	Illnesses characterized by fatigue, lethargy, and weakness, poor appetite and related weight loss, shallow breathing or shortness of breath, and poor resistance to infections.	Tonify and strengthen
Yang	Combination of exterior, hot, and excess conditions characterized by red or ruddy complexion, agitation or hyperactivity, rapid breathing, scant and dark urine, and constipation.	Cool and sedate
Exterior	Illnesses affecting surface of body, and characterized by sudden, acute onset.	Expel or purge; induce perspiration

Principle	Common Symptoms	Treatment
Hot	Illnesses characterized by hot extremities, flushed or reddish complexion, hyperactivity, nervousness, extreme thirst, dark urine, and possible constipation.	Cool and sedate
Excess	Illnesses characterized by feelings of fullness or heaviness, pain, organ obstruction, forceful breathing, possible abdominal distention, tension or restlessness.	Disperse; purge

Additionally, traditional practitioners will also look for another yang-related symptom—false heat—when assessing a patient's illness, because unlike other yang-related conditions that call for cooling herbs, false heat requires warming herbs (usually combined in a yin tonic). False heat symptoms, which occur because of a yin deficiency, include diarrhea and cold extremities, but the person has no aversion to the cold and, in fact, usually has a fever and a flushed or red face.

Moving On to Herbal Treatment

This brief discussion of Oriental Medicine's methods of defining and diagnosing illness is the first but most crucial step on the road to self-treatment. You have probably already recognized some familiar patterns of illness that you, or your loved ones, have experienced, and you now may even be able to reframe several common, everyday ailments from the traditional practitioner's point of view. The case histories that follow discuss three common ailments in everyday language, and demonstrate how diagnosis and treatment are handled from the perspective of Oriental Medicine.

Case History No. 1

John K, thirty-eight, had been plagued by aching and swollen joints that got hot when they were most painful. His right knee was the worst. John is also overweight, so it is reasonable to believe that his knees, which are already taking a lot of abuse because of his extra weight, would also be the first parts of his body to show arthritis-like symptoms. Almost every movement John made was painful, and this caused sleeping difficulties because he couldn't find a comfortable position in which to sleep. Sleeping medications left him tired in the morning anyway, so he stayed away from them. After work, John would always wrap his right knee in ice, which made it feel better and reduced the swelling a little. On occasion, the other knee also acted up, as did his right hand. Besides all this, John had occasional headaches, perspired heavily, even after minor exertion, was always thirsty, and found it difficult to sit still, even though moving the knee hurt. John also suffered from minor skin rashes on occasion, and had a thin, yellow coat on his tongue.

Diagnosis: John was diagnosed both with early-stage arthritis—occasionally accompanied by bouts of sciatica—and with high blood pressure that was exacerbated by his weight problem. In Oriental Medicine terms, he was experiencing symptoms of wind-damp and wind chill, stagnant Qi and Blood, deficient Yin, and rising Heart fire.

Treatment: John received lifestyle and diet counseling. He additionally needed a herbal formula that would relieve pain, dispel wind and damp, invigorate and tonify the Blood, move Qi, nourish Yin, and cool rising Heart fire. Clematis and Stephania (formula no. 12) was the treatment of choice.

❖

Case History No. 2

Marilyn D, forty-eight years old, came to the office because she had had insomnia for the past few years, compounded by menopausal symptoms. She experienced nightmares and night sweating, and regularly woke in the middle of the night—soaked with sweat—with heart palpitations. Marilyn sometimes had ringing in the ears on both sides, and she had been getting more forgetful and having dizzy spells. She always felt thirsty, and she had a red tongue with a slight coating. She had sought help everywhere, from conventional medical doctors to other alternative health-care practitioners, but hormone therapy and other alternative therapies had so far failed.

Diagnosis: Marilyn was diagnosed with early-stage menopausal symptoms that were being greatly exacerbated by a poor diet, little exercise, and a high-stress managerial job that required frequent overtime. Marilyn was also diagnosed with mild anxiety and depression. The latter, together with her menopausal symptoms, were major causes of her insomnia and heart palpitations. In Oriental Medicine terms, she was suffering from an overactive Spirit (Shen), deficient Yin and Blood, and from rising Heart fire.

Treatment: Marilyn received lifestyle and diet counseling. It was also strongly recommended that she follow a mild exercise program, such as t'ai chi chuan. Marilyn additionally needed herbal formulas that would work quickly and safely to calm her spirit, tonifiy her Heart and Blood, nourish her yin, and cool the rising Heart fire. She received Concha Marguerita and Ligustrum (formula no. 14) for two weeks, followed by Ginseng and Zizyphus (formula no. 26).

Case History No. 3

Nancy B, forty-six, a normally robust individual, came to the office suffering with a bad cold that had come on suddenly, two days after watching her daughter play soccer on a windy, rainy spring morning. Nancy had a high fever with a sore throat, a splitting headache that felt better when she pressed both her hands on the sides of her head, and a strong thirst for ice-cold orange juice. She was also coughing, spitting up sticky, yellow phlegm, and had a yellow coating on her tongue.

Diagnosis: Nancy was diagnosed with common seasonal cold symptoms. In Oriental Medicine terms, she was experiencing the effects of a classic external wind-heat injury accompanied by surface (exterior) heat symptoms.

Treatment: Nancy needed a short-term herbal formula that would disperse and clear her toxic wind-heat symptoms, promote sweating, moisten her Lungs, soothe her throat, and stop her coughing. She was given the classic formula, Lonicera and Forsythia (formula no. 31), which every "soccer mom" should have in her medicine cabinet for just these occasions.

The next step on the road to self-treatment is matching the right herbs with the right symptoms. We've already learned that just as illness is essentially yin or yang, so, too, are herbs. But as with everything in traditional Oriental Medicine, herbs are far more than that: they also have specific tastes, natures, and actions—all of which are discussed in greater detail in Chapter Four.

As we move on, then, to herbs and herbal treatment, think about your common, everyday ailments, and remember these simple and general rules:

- If it's *hot*, it should be cooled and/or moistened.
- If it's *cold*, it should be warmed.
- If it's *excessive*, it should be constrained.
- If it's *deficient*, it should be tonified.
- If it's *damp*, it should be dried and/or dispersed.
- If it's *dry*, it should be moistened and/or resolved.

CHAPTER FOUR

Understanding Oriental Medicine: Herbs and Herbal Treatment

Once you have reached a diagnosis of your illness or imbalance, it's time to move on to a course of treatment. In traditional herbal medicine, the treatment of choice will be one or more of Oriental Medicine's famed therapeutic herbal formulas—many of which are discussed in Chapter Seven. But to understand how formulas work, we first need to take a good look at the single herbs that go into them. Those herbs provide the fundamental cornerstones upon which treatment is built.

In Oriental Medicine, relatively few herbs are used alone for medicinal purposes—cinnamon, clove, and gingko biloba being among the more popular exceptions. But the skillful *combination* of herbs, precisely matched for their unique individual properties, is fundamental to the remarkable effectiveness of herbal formulas in treating a variety of ailments and illnesses gently and safely. Learning to combine herbs to make the best possible formulas takes years of training and remains a precise and sophisticated science.

To begin to understand the complexity that underlies herbal formulas, as well as learn how to use formulas most effectively in treatment, we need a fuller appreciation of the individual herbs that make up a formula.

We have already learned that herbs are essentially yin or yang in character, and treat yin or yang imbalances. In addition, herbs possess many other therapeutic properties that make each one unique. Those properties in turn dictate both why certain herbs are combined to treat a specific ailment and how treatment will progress.

The following discussion of the what, why, and how of single herbs will deepen your understanding of the dynamic properties of herbs and serve to introduce the single herbs listed in Chapter Five—all of which are used in the Chinese herbal formulas presented in Chapter Seven.

We begin with a brief look at how plant herbs are grown, harvested, and prepared for sale and shipment, starting with the most basic of questions: what is an herb?

In traditional Oriental Medicine, the term "herb" is generally used to refer to the hundreds of plant, animal, and mineral products pre-scribed preventively or therapeutically by the traditional practitioner. Plant herbs are the most frequently used substances from the traditional Chinese pharmacopoeia—and plant herbs are our primary focus here. But some animal products (for example, oyster shell, earthworm, deer antler) and minerals (magnetitum, dragon bones, talc) are also used in herbal formulas.

The great majority of plant herbs are cultivated on herb farms, and the finest herbs are still grown, harvested, and processed in China, then shipped to herb shops and herbal supply companies worldwide. Different parts of a plant often have different medicinal purposes, and this affects both how and when plants are harvested. The outer parts of the plant—including leaves, twigs, flowers, fruits, and fruit seeds—are believed to work most effectively on the surface of the body or on Organ systems that are closer to the surface (e.g., the Lungs and Heart). These parts of the plant are especially effective in treating external causes of ailments.

Leaves and twigs are usually harvested before a plant's flowers bloom. Flowers are harvested when they have just budded or bloomed. Most fruits are harvested when they have just ripened, but several fruits that are more potent in their immature forms—*Auranti immaturus*, for example—are harvested before ripening. Seeds are harvested just after the fruit has ripened.

The roots, rhizomes, and tubers of a plant, which are usually buried deep in the earth, are believed to most effectively treat internal Organ imbalances that are in turn deeper in the body (the Liver and Spleen systems, for example). Depending on a plant's growing season, roots and tubers are harvested near the end of the growing cycle, in early spring or late autumn.

After herb plants are harvested, they are steam-cleaned to remove dirt,

In Oriental medicine, the *shape* of a plant is also sometimes related to the part of the body it most effectively treats. Ginseng root, for example, which approximates the shape of the human body, is a general-purpose tonic that strengthens and nourishes Qi throughout the body.

The fruit of the walnut, which resembles both the human brain and the Kidney, is used to treat the central nervous system by tonifying (or strengthening) the Qi of the Kidney, the organ that governs proper brain function.

eggs, and parasites. Then they are dried in full sunlight. Next, they are sorted into their various medicinal parts—buds, blooms, seeds, peels, roots, tubers, rhizomes, and bark—and are prepared for storage and shipping. Flower buds, blooms, and seeds are usually packaged whole and labeled accordingly. Roots, tubers, rhizomes, peels, and bark are cut into slices or shavings before being placed into individual, labeled packages. All herbs are stored in dry, cool, and well-ventilated places, and are periodically aired and checked for dampness or spoilage.

Thus the unique therapeutic properties of herbs are preserved throughout harvesting, processing, shipping, and storage. When they arrive at a traditional practitioner's clinic, or at an herbal supply outlet, single herbs are ready to be combined into herbal formulas or prescriptions, according to their characteristic healing properties.

The Healing Properties of Herbs

An herb has four primary healing properties: its *nature, taste, affinity* with specific organs, and its primary *effect* or *action* in the body.

An herb's *nature* is directly related to its yin or yang character: Herbs have *warm* or *hot* (yang), *cool* or *cold* (yin), or *neutral* natures. As we learned earlier, yang (hot) herbs treat yin (cold) conditions, and yin (cold) herbs treat yang (hot) conditions.

Further, yang herbs move upward in the body, to its surface, and are frequently used to treat external conditions of the upper respiratory tract, the skin, and the extremities. Yin herbs move downward in the body, to its interior, and are frequently used to treat internal conditions and organ imbalances.

An herb's nature and healing characteristics may be described as follows:

Nature of Herb	Healing Characteristics
Warm (yang)	Treats cold deficiency conditions. Examples include acoris, agastache, and alpina.
Hot (yang)	Strongly treats cold deficiency conditions. Examples include aconite, cinnamon bark, and fresh ginger.
Cool (yin)	Treats hot excess conditions. Examples include grifola, moutan, and oyster shell.
Cold (yin)	Strongly treats hot excess conditions. Examples include peony rubra, phellodendron, and plantago seed.
Neutral (yin or yang)	Treats cold or hot, deficiency or excess conditions depending on the person and the ailment. Examples include platycodon, poria, and scirpus.

Herbs are also characterized by their *taste—sour*, *bitter*, *sweet* or *bland*, *spicy*, or *salty*. Here, "taste" does not refer to the flavor of the herb itself, but rather to its general therapeutic action on Qi, Blood, Fluids, Phlegm, and internal and external "climate" conditions. Specific tastes have specific healing actions, as shown below.

Taste of Herb	General Therapeutic Action
Sour	Astringes/consolidates/concentrates; sour herbs are often used to treat diarrhea, other excessive bodily discharges, and to concentrate Qi energy. Examples include cornus, schisandra, and ziziphi seed.
Bitter	Eliminates/discharges/moves downward; bitter herbs are often used to treat coughs, constipation, nausea and vomiting, and coronary conditions. Examples include dianthus, gardenia fruit, and gentiana scabra.
Sweet or bland	Harmonizes/nourishes/slows down; sweet and/or bland herbs are often used for their restorative and harmonizing properties and to treat pain. Examples include gastrodia, licorice, and steamed rehmannia.
Spicy	Stimulates/speeds up/moves upward; spicy herbs are often used to improve Blood and Qi circulation. Examples include ginger and ligusticum.
Salty	Softens/breaks up; salty herbs are often used to treat constipation and other abdominal imbalances. Examples include haliotidis, lumbricus, and scrophularia.

Additionally, such *aromatic* herbs as acorus, aquilaria, cardamom seed, and magnolia bark have special therapeutic actions that break up and dislodge persistent phlegm, dispel wind and damp conditions, and restore mental clarity.

Herbs are further characterized by their unique *affinity* with specific Organs in the body, or, as we illustrate in this book, with specific Organ-related meridians that the herbs "enter." In general:

- Sour herbs have an affinity for the Liver and Gallbladder
- Bitter herbs have an affinity for the Heart and Small Intestine
- Sweet or bland herbs have an affinity for the Stomach and Spleen
- Spicy herbs have an affinity for the Lungs and Large Intestine
- Salty herbs have an affinity for the Kidneys and Bladder

Herbs are also characterized by their specific *effects* or *actions* in the body. Generally, herbs *dispel, astringe, purge,* or *tonify* imbalances of Qi, Blood, fluids, phlegm, and the external or internal climate-related imbalances of wind, heat, cold, dryness, and dampness.

Effect of Herb	*General Action*
Dispels	Moves, relaxes, and/or redistributes where there is accumulation, stagnation, sluggishness, or spasms. Examples include alismatis, atractylodes, and cinnamon twig.
Astringes	Consolidates, holds, restrains, and/or tightens where there is leaking, discharge, or excessive elimination. Examples include astragalus, cornus, and pseudoginseng.
Purges	Eliminates, expels, and/or detoxifies where there is obstruction, chronic stagnation, or "poison" (toxicity). Examples include dianthus, magnolia bark, and stephania.
Tonifies	Nourishes, strengthens, enhances, supports, calms, and/or protects where there is deficiency and "emptyness." Examples include angelica root, dioscorea, and ligustrum.

The following chart illustrates the unique healing effects of over eighty major Chinese herbs. All of these herbs are described in detail in Chapter Five. The numbers in parentheses refer to their numerical listing in that chapter.

HEALING EFFECTS OF MAJOR SINGLE HERBS

Herbs that dispel external wind, cold, heat, and damp

Angelica Dahurica (12)
Asarum (19)
Bupleurum (29)
Carthamus Flower (34)
Cinnamon Twig (39)
Ephedra (61)
Magnolia Flower (95)
Perilla Leaf (107)
Pueraria (117)
Schizonepeta (125)

Herbs that dispel internal heat/damp and purge fire

Anemarrhena (10)
Bamboo Leaf (27)
Coptis (46)
Forsythia Fruit (65)
Gardenia Fruit (68)
Gentiana Scabra (72)
Isatidis (79)
Lonicera Flower (87)
Lycium (90)
Moutan (98)
Nelumbinus Stamen (100)
Peony Alba (104)
Phellodendron (108)
Prunella (114)
Scrophularia (127)
Scutellaria (128)
Sophora (131)

Herbs that astringe

Cornus (48)
Schisandra (124)

Herbs that dispel internal cold

Aconite (2)
Cinnamon Bark (38)
Evodia (63)
Fennel (64)
Ginger (fresh) (94)

Herbs that dispel excess fluids

Akebia (5)
Alismatis (7)
Coix (45)
Dioscoria (54)
Plantago Seed (110)
Poria (114)
Talc (133)

Herbs that break up and expel phlegm

Apricot Seed (15)
Arisaema (18)
Fritillaria (67)
Inula (78)
Pinellia (109)
Platycodon (111)

Herbs that promote blood circulation

Achyranthes (1)
Carthamus Flower (34)
Curcuma (50)
Ligusticum (83)
Pseudoginseng (116)
Salvia (121)
Sophora (131)

Herbs that tonify Qi

Astragalus (21)
Atractylodes Alba (23)
Citri Immaturi (41)
Citrus Peel (43)
Codonopsis (44)
Cyperus (52)
Dioscoria (54)
Ginseng (75)
Licorice (82)
Saussurea (123)
Ziziphi Fruit (138)

Herbs that tonify yang

Alpina (8)
Cistanches (40)
Cornu Cervi (47)
Dipsacus (55)
Eucommia Bark (62)
Tribuli (134)

Herbs that tonify yin

Eclipta (60)
Lycium (91)

Herbs that tonify blood

Angelica Sinensis (13)
Longan (86)
Polygonum Multiflorum (113)
Rehmannia (steamed) (119)

Herbs that calm and sedate

Dragon Bone (58)
Magnetitum (93)
Oyster Shell (103)
Polygala (112)
Ziziphi Seed (139)

Putting It All Together: How Herbs Are Combined

Generally, every Chinese formula is constructed around one or two primary herbs that are the therapeutic heart of the formula, and a group of secondary herbs that function synergistically to support the primary herbs.

Primary herbs target the specific ailment or imbalance and are the most potent herbs in the formula. Secondary herbs have three functions. One or more is therapeutically similar to the primary herbs and serves to enhance those herbs' healing benefits and ensure the overall effectiveness of the formula. Another group of secondary herbs functions both to offset unwanted side effects that would inhibit the therapeutic action of the formula, and/or mitigate any toxicities in the other herbs in the formula. And a final group of secondary herbs serves to strengthen and nourish the body while it is healing, as well as harmonize the effects of the other herbs by ensuring that their healing benefits are quickly and thoroughly distributed throughout the body.

Thus a warm and sweet herb whose primary function, for example, is to tonify and nourish deficient Blood may be secondarily supported by a cool and bitter herb whose function is to stop bleeding and increase circulation. Likewise, a warm and bitter herb used to treat fluid retention by astringing (drying up) excessive internal dampness may be supported by a neutral and bland herb that nourishes and harmonizes the body and offsets dehydration. Similarly, herbs whose primary function is to tonify and nourish Qi and Blood are supported by herbs that move Qi and Blood through the body. And potent purging herbs that forcefully rid the body of excess toxins, wastes, and fluids are supported by tonifying and nourishing herbs that protect the body from being overtaxed.

The following chart aptly illustrates the unique dynamics of combining herbs therapeutically. Listed are ten of the single herbs discussed in Chapter Five by their nature, taste, action, and effects in the body, together with the common ailments that they treat—described in conventional Western and traditional Oriental Medicine terms. When variously combined, these herbs become the ingredients of two of Oriental Medicine's most renowned formulas—Rehmannia Six and Tang Gui Four. And while the formulas share one famous herb—rehmannia—they have singularly different effects.

Rehmannia Six is a renowned general tonic that tonifies and nourishes Blood and yin and primarily treats internal heat and dry imbal-

HERBAL PROPERTIES AND ACTIONS IN REHMANNIA SIX FORMULA* AND TANG-GUI FOUR FORMULA**

Herb	Nature/Taste	Organ Affinity	Action	Effect	OM Symptoms	Conventional Symptoms	OM Treatment
Rehmannia (steamed)	Warm/Sweet	Liver, Kidneys, Heart	Nourishes and harmonizes	Tonifies Blood	Blood and yin deficiencies	Dizziness; palpitations; insomnia; irregular menstruation; night sweats; lower-back pain	Tonify Blood and nourish yin
Alisma	Cool/Sweet, bland	Kidneys, Bladder	Nourishes and slows down	Disperses and moves moisture	Internal heat-damp imbalances	Difficulty in urination; blood in urine; pelvic infections; diarrhea; leukorrhea; herpes; abdominal bloating; kidney stones	Promote urination; drain dampness; nourish yin
Cornus	Warm/Sour	Kidneys, Lungs, Liver	Astringes	Astringes and consolidates moisture; concentrates Qi	Excess internal damp; deficient Qi	Excessive menstruation; copious sweating; pain in lower back and knees; dizziness; poor hearing	Astringe essence and dampness; stablize Kidneys and Liver
Dioscoria	Neutral/Sweet	Kidneys, Lungs, Spleen	Nourishes and harmonizes	Nourishes and harmonizes Organs; consolidates Qi	Internal deficiency	Chronic weakness; fatigue; diarrhea; excessive sweating; poor appetite; asthma with cough	Nourish Kidneys and Lungs; tonify Spleen and Stomach

Poria Cocos	Neutral/Sweet, bland	Heart, Spleen, Lungs	Nourishes and harmonizes	Disperses moisture	Deficient heat and internal damp	Fluid congestion and retention	Promote urination and astringe dampness; disperse phlegm; calm spirit
Moutan	Cool/Acrid, bitter	Heart, Liver, Kidneys	Dispels, moves, and drains	Moves Blood; Clears heat and fire; dispels congealed Blood	Stagnant Blood; internal heat and fire	Missing or irregular menstrual periods; abnormal bleeding; swelling; masses, and lumps; high fever; skin eruptions	Clear heat and cool Blood; clear fire; invigorate Blood and dispel stagnation; reduce swelling
Peony Alba	Cool/Bitter, sour	Liver, Spleen	Astringes, eliminates, and moves Qi	Tonifies Blood; consolidates Qi; preserves yin	Internal heat/Blood imbalance with spasms and pain	Excessive bleeding; muscle spasms; poor circulation	Nourish Blood; stop bleeding; restrain yin; adjust Nutritive and Protective Qi; promote circulation
Angelica	Warm/Sweet, acrid, bitter	Spleen, Kidneys	Astringes and eliminates damp; moves Qi downward	Tonifies Blood	Deficient heat; deficient or stagnant Blood; internal damp	Irregular menstruation with dry skin and headache	Tonify and invigorate Blood; moisten intestines and move stool; regulate menses
Ligusticum	Warm/Acrid or bitter	Liver, Gallbladder, Pericardium	Astringes and expels damp; moves Qi	Moves and invigorates Blood	External wind injury; stagnant Qi; stagnant Blood	Menstrual irregularity; headaches; chest and rib pain	Expel wind; invigorate Blood; move Qi; alleviate pain

*Rehmannia (steamed), Alisma, Cornus, Dioscoria, Poria Cocos, and Moutan are found in Rehmannia Six Formula.

**Rehmannia (steamed), Peony Alba, Angelica, and Ligusticum are found in Tang-Gui Four Formula.

ances—hence the addition of the two cooler herbs. Tang Gui Four is famed for its effectiveness in treating menstrual irregularities, a condition of stagnant Blood and Qi and internal cold (deficient heat)—thus the appearance of warming and neutral herbs, and herbs that move both Qi and Blood.

Each of the 139 herbs featured in Chapter Five has its own unique healing actions and benefits. And all these herbs appear, in a variety of combinations, in the herbal formulas that are at the heart of this home guide to Chinese herbal medicine. Reading through the descriptions of the single herbs will give you a fuller understanding of the herbal formulas that follow. Then you can confidently move on to choosing the right herbs for the right ailments.

CHAPTER FIVE

A Chinese Pharmacopoeia: 139 Healing Herbs

The healing herbs described in this chapter are the ones most frequently used in Chinese herbal formulas. Here they are listed numerically in alphabetical order by their common English or Latin names. Each entry also displays the Latin plant name, followed by the pinyin Mandarin name in italics, together with an illustration of the corresponding Chinese ideogram for the herb. The ideograms are especially useful to have if you buy herbs from a neighborhood herbal shop where language barriers may exist. Showing the ideograms for the herbs you want to buy will ensure your getting the proper ingredients for your formula. Any alternate English names for the herb are also listed.

The part of the plant most often used in herbal formulas is also displayed, as are the herb's primary healing properties, including its nature, taste, and Organ affinity (listed here as "Meridians Entered").

Under "Common Usages" you will find a brief description of the general symptoms the herb treats, described in conventional medical terms, with the corresponding Oriental Medical ("OM") diagnoses shown where appropriate in parentheses and italics.

The herb's traditional effects or actions in the body are described under "Traditional Usages and Functions" in classic Oriental Medicine language.

The names of the formulas in which a herb is used are shown under

A FRIENDLY WARNING!

It is a common fallacy to believe that everything natural and cultivated from the earth is safe and beneficent. This simply isn't true. Remember, the beloved Emperor Sheng Nung, China's patron saint of herbal medicine, poisoned himself many times before he wrote his renowned drug compendium, *The Herbal Classic of the Divine Plowman*. Approach the use of herbs with an open mind and open heart, but also with respect and caution.

Herbs are medicine, and thus they should be used wisely and moderately. Indeed, while the single herbs described here are generally safe when used in formulas, we discourage their use alone, and in fact, we give no dosage information here just to underscore that precaution. (Gingko biloba is a notable exception.)

We encourage you to visit a traditional Oriental Medicine practitioner at some point in your journey to good health. He or she will do a thorough assessment of your state of health, work with you to outline specific goals for overall wellness, and monitor your recovery, making adjustments in herbal treatment as needed.

In the case of serious and chronic diseases, we also strongly encourage you to work under the supervision of a traditional practitioner, and to take advantage of the best that both traditional and conventional medicine have to offer.

"Common Formulas Used In," and the formulas themselves may be found, in alphabetical order, in Chapter Seven.

Any other interesting characteristics of the herb or special instructions about its use will be found under "Remarks."

Finally, prohibitions and cautions against a particular herb's use will be found under "Cautions in Use."

1. Achyranthes

牛膝

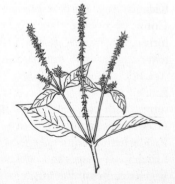

Latin Plant Name: Achyranthes Bidentata
Pinyin Mandarin Name: *Niu Xi*
Common English Name: Achyranthes
Part of Plant Used: Root
Nature: Neutral
Taste: Bitter, sour
Meridians Entered: Liver, Kidneys

Common Usages: Most often used in formulas that strengthen the back and knees *(OM: tonifies the Kidneys; reins in Liver Yang; moves Blood and dampness);* for trauma, boils, painful or absent menses, and tendon and bone disruptions *(OM: for lower-body Blood stasis and stagnation);* for nosebleeds, bleeding gums, and toothaches *(OM: for deficient Yin with Blood heat);* for dizziness, headaches, or blurred vision *(OM: for deficient Yin with Blood heat and rising Liver Yang);* and may also be used for Kidney stones and painful urination with blood.

Traditional Usages and Functions: Invigorates Blood; expels congealed Blood; strengthens sinews and bones and benefits joints; clears damp heat in Lower Burner; induces downward movement of Blood.

Common Formulas Used In: Clematis and Stephania; Leonuris and Achyranthes; Tu-Huo and Eucommia.

Remarks: Often used in a wine preparation for its tonifying actions.

Cautions in Use: Do not use during pregnancy; with diarrhea from deficient Spleen; with excessive menstruation; or with leakage of sperm.

2. Aconite

附 子

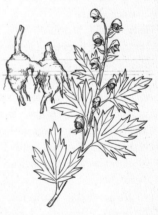

Latin Plant Name: Aconitum Carmichaeli Preparata
Pinyin Mandarin Name: *Fu Zi*
Common English Name: Aconite
Part of Plant Used: Prepared root
Nature: Hot, poisonous
Taste: Acrid, sweet
Meridians Entered: Heart, Spleen, Kidneys
Common Usages: This herb is used in formulas that stimulate the metabolism and tonify the heart muscle *(OM: "wakens the yang," produces heat, moves water).*

Traditional Usages and Functions: Restores devastated Yang; warms Kidney Fire; strengthens yang; warms Kidney and Spleen; expels cold; warms and opens the channels; alleviates pain.

Common Formulas Used In: Rehmannia Eight.

Processing Required: Aconite is generally prepared to remove its toxicity.

Remarks: Aconite is used in small doses since it is a strong preparation.

It is rarely used alone, except topically, and is usually combined with other warming herbs.

Cautions in Use: Do not use during pregnancy. Although there are usually warnings of its toxicity, aconite's prepared forms are only mildly toxic and in formulas are considered quite safe. If you find yourself feeling too warm while taking a formula containing aconite, just discontinue the formula or remove the aconite. Aconite should not be used where there is a Yin deficiency with heat.

3. Acorus

菖蒲

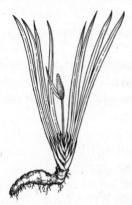

Latin Plant Name: Acori Graminei
Pinyin Mandarin Name: *Chang Pu* or *Shi Chang Pu*
Common English Name: Sweet Flag
Part of Plant Used: Root
Nature: Warm
Taste: Acrid, aromatic
Meridians Entered: Heart, Liver, Spleen

Common Usages: Most often used in formulas to treat fainting or seizures *(OM: for dampness and excess phlegm blocking orifices of the Heart)*; and for poor memory, lack of clarity of thought, ear infections, anorexia, bloating, and parasites.

Traditional Usages and Functions: This aromatic plant strongly stimulates movement within the body to expel phlegm and dampness. Opens the orifices; vaporizes phlegm; harmonizes the Middle Burner; transforms turbid dampness.

Common Formulas Used In: Cerebral Tonic Pills; Concha Marguerita and Ligustrum.

Cautions in Use: Use with caution where there is deficient Yin. Phlegm often is poorly metabolized yin, and the herb may "vaporize" some of the yin with the phlegm. This, in turn, can intensify Yin-deficiency signs such as false heat. Also use cautiously with deficient heat, or if there is irritability with excessive sweating, vomiting of blood, or leakage of sperm.

4. Agastache

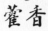

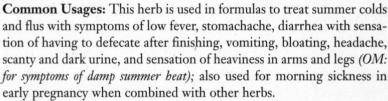

Latin Plant Name: Agastaches seu Pogostemi

Pinyin Mandarin Name: *Huo Xiang*

Part of Plant Used: Whole plant is used, but leaves are the most aromatic

Common English Name: Patchouli

Nature: Warm

Taste: Acrid, aromatic

Meridians Entered: Lung, Spleen, Stomach

Common Usages: This herb is used in formulas to treat summer colds and flus with symptoms of low fever, stomachache, diarrhea with sensation of having to defecate after finishing, vomiting, bloating, headache, scanty and dark urine, and sensation of heaviness in arms and legs *(OM: for symptoms of damp summer heat);* also used for morning sickness in early pregnancy when combined with other herbs.

Traditional Usages and Functions: Transforms dampness; balances the Middle Burner and stops vomiting; helps throw off attacking pathogens by causing sweating.

Common Formulas Used In: Agastache.

Remarks: Agastache is added last when preparing raw herbs for drinking since it has aromatic qualities that will dissipate with long boiling.

Cautions in Use: This aromatic plant strongly stimulates movement within the body, and as a result it must be used carefully when there is deficient yin with heat signs or if there is Stomach heat.

5. Akebia

木通

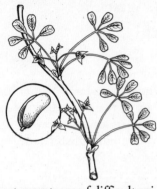

Latin Plant Name: Akebiae Caulis
Pinyin Mandarin Name: *Mu Tong*
Common English Name: Akebia
Part of Plant Used: Stem (caulis)
Nature: Cool
Taste: Bitter
Meridians Entered: Heart, Small
Intestine, Bladder

Common Usages: This herb is used to treat symptoms of difficult urination, insomnia, absent menstruation, sore tongue and throat, joint
pains, poor circulation, and deficient lactation *(OM: internal damp heat).*
Traditional Usages and Functions: Promotes urination and drains
heat from the Heart via the Small Intestine; promotes lactation and
unblocks blood vessels.
Common Formulas Used In: Dianthus; Gentiana.
Cautions in Use: Do not use during pregnancy. Use with extreme caution where there are deficient-Yin conditions since akebia strongly promotes urination.

6. Albizza

合歡皮

Latin Plant Name: Albizza Julibrissin
Pinyin Mandarin Name: *He Huan Pi*
Common English Name: Mimosa Tree
Part of Plant Used: Bark
Nature: Neutral
Taste: Sweet
Meridians Entered: Heart, Liver,
Spleen, Lungs

Common Usages: Most often used in formulas to build and repair
fractured bones and help speed the healing process *(OM: increases blood
circulation and calms the spirit);* also used to treat symptoms of insomnia,
emotional imbalance, excessive worry, fright, nightmares, and paranoia
(OM: calms the spirit); and may be useful for Lung abscesses with expectoration of blood with phlegm.

Traditional Usages and Functions: Calms the Spirit; invigorates the Blood; alleviates pain; dissipates abscesses.
Common Formulas Used In: Concha Marguerita and Ligustrum.
Cautions in Use: None.

7. Alismatis
澤瀉

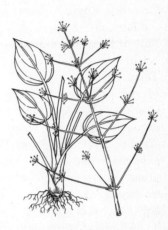

Latin Plant Name: Alismatis Plantago-Aquaticae
Pinyin Mandarin Name: *Ze Xie*
Common English Name: Water Plantain
Part of Plant Used: Tuberous stem (bulb)
Nature: Cold
Taste: Sweet, bland
Meridians Entered: Kidneys, Bladder
Common Usages: This herb is most often used in formulas for its ability to gently promote urination; also used to treat blood in the urine, difficulty in urination, diarrhea, thirst, and phlegm retention; may also be used for pelvic infections, leukorrhea (mucousy vaginal discharge), herpes, abdominal bloating, kidney stones, and diabetic syndrome.
Traditional Usages and Functions: For urinary-tract heat-damp imbalances without the strong yin-injuring effect of many other herbs and diuretics that drain dampness.
Common Formulas Used In: Anemarrhena, Phellodendron, and Rehmannia Eight; Immortal Long Life Pill; Gentiana; Hoelen Five; Rehmannia and Dogwood Fruit; Rehmannia and Magnetitum; Rehmannia Eight; Rehmannia Six.
Cautions in Use: Long-term usage of alismatis can irritate the intestines. Do not use with deficient Kidney Yang or damp cold with leakage of sperm or with leukorrhea.

8. Alpina

益智仁

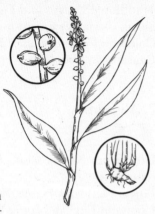

Latin Plant Name: Alpiniae Oxyphyllae
Pinyin Mandarin Name: *Yi Zhi Ren*
Common English Name: Black
Cardamom
Part of Plant Used: Fruit
Nature: Warm
Taste: Acrid
Meridians Entered: Spleen, Kidneys
Common Usages: Most often used in
formulas to improve digestion and treat
diarrhea *(OM: strengthens Yang of Spleen and Stomach and treats cold
imbalances)*; also used for night urination and sperm leakage; frequent
urination, drooling, and abdominal pain *(OM: treats Yang deficiency with
symptoms of core coldness and inability to get warm; builds Kidney Yang and
helps body retain or astringe fluids; calms the spirit)*.
Traditional Usages and Functions: Warms the Kidneys; retains
Essence and holds in urine; warms the Spleen; stops diarrhea.
Common Formulas Used In: Hoelen and Polyporus.
Cautions in Use: Do not use in cases of sperm leakage or leukorrhea
with strong signs of heat.

9. Amber

琥珀

Latin Plant Name: Succinum
Pinyin Mandarin Name: *Hu Po*
Common English Name: Amber
Part of Plant Used: Amber is the
petrified resin of trees buried
underground for years; the tree is long
extinct.
Nature: Neutral
Taste: Sweet
Meridians Entered: Heart, Liver, Small Intestine, Bladder
Common Usages: This herb is used in many liniments for its antisep-
tic and skin-healing properties. It is also used in many formulas for its

ability to sedate and calm the Spirit, invigorate and move Blood, and promote healing, which makes it particularly useful for individuals—especially children—who are recovering from an injury where there is Blood stagnation and sleep anxiety. Amber is also very useful for post-birth abdominal pain due to Blood stagnation.

Traditional Usages and Functions: Sedates and calms the Spirit; promotes urination; invigorates Blood; promotes menstruation; reduces swelling and promotes healing.

Common Formulas Used In: Cerebral Tonic Pills; Leonuris and Achyranthes.

Cautions in Use: Do not use with heat signs due to Yin deficiency.

10. Anemarrhena

知母

Latin Plant Name: Anemarrhenae Asphodeloidis
Pinyin Mandarin Name: *Zhi Mu*
Common English Name: Anemarrhena
Part of Plant Used: Root
Nature: Cold
Taste: Bitter
Meridians Entered: Lung, Stomach, Kidney
Common Usages: This herb is often used in formulas to treat coughs with yellow phlegm, fever, dry stools, and other internal heat conditions; and to treat diabetics with symptoms of irritability and fever *(OM: Yin-deficiency heat symptoms)*.

Traditional Usages and Functions: Clears heat and quells fire; nurtures yin and moistens dry conditions; drains heat in the Lower Burner; generates fluids and clears heat.

Common Formulas Used In: Anemarrhena, Phellodendron, and Rehmannia; Xanthium and Magnolia.

Cautions in Use: Do not use if there is watery diarrhea *(OM: deficient Spleen)*.

11. Angelica Du Huo
獨活

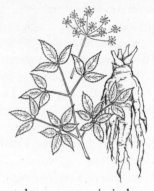

Latin Plant Name: Angelica Pubescens
Pinyin Mandarin Name: *Du Huo*
Common English Name: Angelica
Du Huo
Part of Plant Used: Root
Nature: Mildly warm
Taste: Bitter, acrid
Meridians Entered: Kidney, Bladder
Common Usages: This herb is used in formulas to treat pain in lower back and legs due to exposure to wind, cold, and dampness *(OM: external wind, external cold, and external damp conditions)*, and to treat symptoms of headaches from colds, pain in lower abdomen, and sore knees and lower back *(OM: external wind and external damp)*.
Traditional Usages and Functions: Expels wind dampness and alleviates pain; also combined with other herbs to treat Blood stagnation.
Common Formulas Used In: Tian Man and Eucommia; Tu-Huo and Loranthus.
Cautions in Use: Do not use with deficient-Yin heat signs or with deficient Blood with obstruction.

12. Angelica Dahurica
白芷

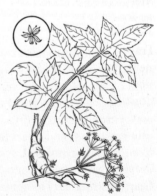

Latin Plant Name: Angelica Dahurica
Pinyin Mandarin Name: *Bai Zhi*
Common English Name: Angelica
Dahurica
Part of Plant Used: Root
Nature: Warm
Taste: Acrid
Meridians Entered: Lungs, Stomach
Common Usages: This herb is most often used in formulas to treat headaches or toothaches; also used to treat symptoms of upper-body congestion, sinus headache, and acute acne and itching *(OM: strong external wind-cold injury)*. Also used for its drying effects in treating symptoms of leukorrhea with white or pink vaginal discharge.

Traditional Usages and Functions: Expels wind and alleviates pain; reduces swelling and expels pus; expels dampness and alleviates discharge; opens nasal passages.

Common Formulas Used In: Agastache; Clematis and Stephania; Cnidium and Tea; Corydalis Tuber; Xanthium and Magnolia.

Cautions in Use: This herb is very drying and should be used carefully where there are sores that are already draining well, or where there is a Blood or Yin deficiency.

13. Angelica Sinensis

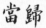 當歸

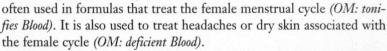

Latin Plant Name: Angelica Sinensis
Pinyin Mandarin Name: *Tang Gui*
Common English Name: Angelica Sinensis
Part of Plant Used: Root
Nature: Warm
Taste: Sweet, acrid, bitter
Meridians Entered: Spleen, Kidneys
Common Usages: This herb regulates the female reproductive organs and is most often used in formulas that treat the female menstrual cycle *(OM: tonifies Blood)*. It is also used to treat headaches or dry skin associated with the female cycle *(OM: deficient Blood)*.

Traditional Usages and Functions: Tonifies Blood and regulates menses; invigorates and harmonizes Blood; moistens Intestines and moves stool.

Common Formulas Used In: Angelica; Bupleurum and Tang Gui; Cerebral Tonic Pills; Cimicafuga; Clematis and Stephania; Gentiana; Ginseng and Astragalus; Ginseng and Longan; Ginseng and Tang Gui; Ginseng and Zizyphus; Leonuris and Achyranthes; Pseudoginseng and Dragon Blood; Qiang-Huo and Turmeric; Rehmannia and Dogwood Fruit; Tang Gui and Gardenia; Tang Gui and Ginseng Eight; Tang Gui and Indigo; Tang Gui Four; Tu-Huo and Loranthus.

Remarks: Generally only the root of the plant is used and different parts of the root are said to have different actions. The head of the root is supposed to be the most tonifying, while the tail is said to move the Blood more strongly. The root is sold in slices that have been steamed in wine.

Cautions in Use: Use with caution where there is diarrhea, or where there is bloating due to dampness, or signs of Yin deficiency with heat.

14. Antelope Horn

羚羊角

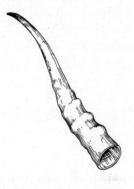

Latin Plant Name: Cornu Antelopis (Saiga Tatarica)
Pinyin Mandarin Name: Ling Yang Jiao
Common English Name: Antelope Horn
Part of Plant Used: Horn
Nature: Cold
Taste: Salty
Meridians Entered: Liver, Heart
Common Usages: This herb is most often used in formulas that treat strokes and seizures and other severe heat-related imbalances *(OM: acute heat imbalances; internal wind imbalances; rising Liver Yang)*.
Traditional Usages and Functions: Pacifies Liver; extinguishes wind; quells heat and detoxifies fire poison; clears damp heat.
Common Formulas Used In: Leonuris and Achyranthes.
Cautions in Use: None.

15. Apricot Seed

杏仁

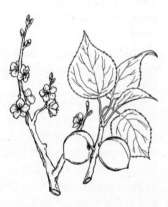

Latin Plant Name: Pruni Armeniacae
Pinyin Mandarin Name: *Xing Ren* or *Ku Xing Ren*
Common English Name: Apricot Seed
Part of Plant Used: Mature seed
Nature: Warm
Taste: Bitter, slightly poisonous
Meridians Entered: Lungs, Large Intestine
Common Usages: This herb is most often used in formulas to treat coughs or wheezing; may also be used to treat constipation *(OM: for heat or cold imbalances, with other herbal ingredients accordingly adjusted to balance formula)*.

Traditional Usages and Functions: Relieves coughs and stops wheezing; moistens Intestines and moves stool.

Remarks: This herb is high in plant oils, which is said to be the chief reason for its laxative properties.

Common Formulas Used In: Apricot Seed and Fritillaria; Apricot Seed and Linum; Clematis and Stephania; Ma Huang.

Cautions in Use: Use cautiously. This herb can be toxic in higher doses: adult toxic dose is fifty to sixty kernels; children's toxic dose is ten kernels.

16. Aquilaria

沉香

Latin Plant Name: Aquilariae Agallocha
Pinyin Mandarin Name: *Chen Xiang*
Common English Name: Aquilaria
Part of Plant Used: Heart of the woody part of the plant
Nature: Warm
Taste: Acrid, bitter, aromatic
Meridians Entered: Lungs, Stomach, Spleen, Kidneys

Common Usages: This herb is most often used in formulas to help foster proper digestive function; may also be used in asthma formulas *(OM: dispels cold; strengthens Kidney Qi)*.

Traditional Usages and Functions: Moves Qi and alleviates pain; reverses rebellious Qi; aids Kidneys in grasping Qi; supplements yang and disperses cold.

Common Formulas Used In: Bupleurum, Inula, and Cyperus; Leonuris and Achyranthes.

Cautions in Use: As with other aromatic herbs, care must be taken where deficient Qi is present. Also use cautiously where there is deficient Yin with heat signs.

17. Areca Husk

大腹皮

Latin Plant Name: Arecae Catechu
Pinyin Mandarin Name: *Da Fu Pi*
Common English Name: Betel Husk
Part of Plant Used: Dried fruit husk of betel nut
Nature: Slightly warm
Taste: Acrid
Meridians Entered: Spleen, Stomach, Large
Intestine, Small Intestine
Common Usages: This herb is most often used in
formulas that treat bloating and congestion in the digestive tract, regulate digestion, promote urination, and treat general edema *(OM: for stagnant Qi and dampness)*. May also be used in some formulas to treat worms due to its paralyzing effect on tapeworms in the bowel.
Traditional Usages and Functions: Moves Qi and reduces stagnation; expels dampness; promotes urination and moves dampness.
Common Formulas Used In: Agastache.
Cautions in Use: Use cautiously where there is Qi deficiency.

18. Arisaema

天南星

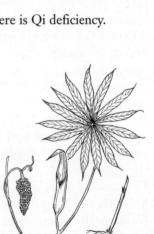

Latin Plant Name: Arisaematis
(Arisaema Amurense)
Pinyin Mandarin Name: *Tain Nan Xing*
Common English Name: Jack-in-the-
Pulpit
Part of Plant Used: Root
Nature: Warm
Taste: Bitter, acrid, poisonous
Meridians Entered: Lungs, Liver,
Spleen
Common Usages: This herb is used in formulas to treat excess moisture (fluid) and phlegm congestion *(OM: dampness)* where there is also nerve and joint involvement, with symptoms of dizziness, numb extremities, facial paralysis (Bell's palsy), spasms of the hands or feet, insomnia, and stroke or seizures *(OM: internal wind imbalances)*. May also be used

solely to help expectorate phlegm. Topically, this herb is useful for sores, ulcerations, and general swelling from trauma or bursitis.

Traditional Usages and Functions: Dries dampness and expels phlegm; disperses wind phlegm in the channels; reduces swelling and alleviates pain.

Common Formulas Used In: Cerebral Tonic Pills.

Remarks: Arisaema is fairly toxic, so its processed version is most often used for internal use, and the unprocessed form is used topically.

Cautions in Use: Do not use during pregnancy. Arisaema is very drying: do not use with deficient Yin, dry phlegm, or hot, dry Lungs.

19. Asarum

細辛

Latin Plant Name: Asarum Sieboldi
(Asari cum Radice)
Pinyin Mandarin Name: *Xi Xin*
Common English Name: Chinese Wild
Ginger
Part of Plant Used: Whole
Nature: Warm
Taste: Acrid
Meridians Entered: Lungs, Spleen,
Kidneys

Common Usages: This herb has warming and dispersing qualities and is used most often in formulas to treat the congestion of sinusitis *(OM: internal cold-damp symptoms and stagnation)* with accompanying headaches, toothaches, fever, and chills; to break up the copious clear or white phlegm of asthma with cough *(OM: internal Lung-cold symptoms)*; and to treat arthritis, especially when the ribs are affected *(OM: internal damp-cold symptoms and Qi stagnation)*.

Traditional Usages and Functions: Repels pathogens; alleviates pain due to wind; warms Lungs and transforms phlegm; opens up areas of stagnation. Asarum is said to direct the action of other herbs to the Heart and Kidney meridians, especially in the arms and chest.

Common Formulas Used In: Cnidium and Tea; Tu-Huo and Loranthus.

Cautions in Use: Do not use during pregnancy. Do not use with Yin-deficiency headaches or with cough due to heat in the Lungs (yellow phlegm). Use only in small quantities.

20. Asparagus

天門冬

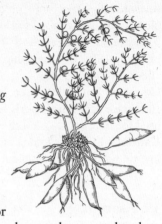

Latin Plant Name: Asparagi
Cochinchinensis
Pinyin Mandarin Name: *Tian Men Dong*
Common English Name: Chinese
Asparagus
Part of Plant Used: Root
Nature: Cold
Taste: Sweet, bitter
Meridians Entered: Lungs, Kidneys
Common Usages: This herb is used for
its moistening effects in formulas that treat dry coughs or coughs where
there is thick sputum streaked with blood; dry skin; excessive thirst; and
the early stages of the "Thirsting and Wasting Syndrome" of diabetes
(*OM: internal fire and dryness symptoms of excess yang; deficient Lung Yin;
deficient Kidney Yin*).
Traditional Usages and Functions: Nourishes the Yin and clears heat;
moistens the Lungs and nourishes the Kidneys.
Common Formulas Used In: Ginseng and Zizyphus.
Cautions in Use: Do not use where there is deficiency-cold diarrhea.

21. Astragalus

黄耆

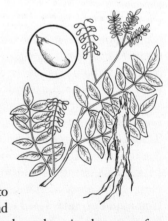

Latin Plant Name: Astragali
Pinyin Mandarin Name: Huang Qi
Common English Name: Milk Vetch
Root
Part of Plant Used: Root
Nature: Slightly warm
Taste: Sweet
Meridians Entered: Spleen, Lungs
Common Usages: Most often used to
stimulate immune-system function and
enhance or speed healing and/or draining where there is edema, pus for-
mation, or chronic ulceration (*OM: treats deficiency of Qi and most other defi-
cient conditions except deficient-yin syndromes with heat signs*); also used to treat

debilitating excessive sweating with accompanying weakness *(OM: tonifies Qi and helps close pores).*

Traditional Usages and Functions: Tonifies Spleen and benefits Qi; raises the Yang Qi of the Spleen and Stomach; strengthens the exterior (the body's first line of defense) and stops sweating; promotes urination and removes edema; promotes healing and discharge of pus; tonifies Qi and Blood.

Common Formulas Used In: Ginseng and Astragalus; Ginseng and Longan; Ginseng and Tang Gui Ten; Stephania and Astragalus.

Remarks: Astragalus is renowned for its superb immune-enhancing properties. Entire books have been written on this herb alone.

Cautions in Use: None.

22. Atractylodes
苍术

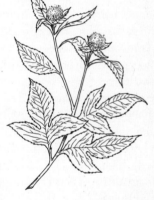

Latin Plant Name: Atractylodes Lancea
Pinyin Mandarin Name: *Cang Zhu*
Common English Name: Atractylodes
Part of Plant Used: Root
Nature: Warm
Taste: Acrid, bitter, aromatic
Meridians Entered: Spleen, Stomach
Common Usages: This herb is most often used in formulas that treat rheumatic arthritis with symptoms of dull pain in the joints, poor appetite, fatigue, and nausea. *(OM: internal damp conditions; deficient Spleen).* It is also useful in treating the night blindness caused by vitamin-A deficiency.

Traditional Usages and Functions: Dries dampness and strengthens the Spleen; expels wind dampness; clears dampness in the Lower Burner; causes sweating and expels pathogens.

Common Formulas Used In: Clematis and Stephania; Cyperus and Ligusticum.

Cautions in Use: Avoid use in conditions of excessive sweating due to deficient Qi or deficient Yin with heat signs.

23. Atractylodes Alba
白术

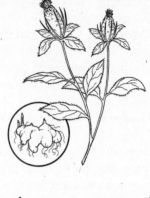

Latin Plant Name: Atractylodis Macrocephalae
Pinyin Mandarin Name: *Bai Zhu*
Common English Name: White Atractylodes
Part of Plant Used: Root
Nature: Warm
Taste: Bitter, sweet
Meridians Entered: Spleen, Stomach
Common Usages: Most often used in formulas to treat symptoms of edema with decreased urination, spontaneous sweating, diarrhea, fatigue, poor appetite, and sometimes vomiting *(OM: for deficiency conditions causing poor metabolism of moisture in body)*; and has been used in formulas to prevent miscarriage *(OM: due to Spleen deficiency)*.
Traditional Usages and Functions: Tonifies Spleen and benefits Qi; strengthens Spleen and dries dampness; stabilizes exterior and stops sweating.
Common Formulas Used In: Agastache; Angelica; Bupleurum and Tang Gui; Ginseng and Astragalus; Ginseng and Atractylodes; Ginseng and Longan; Ginseng and Tang Gui Ten; Hoelen Five; Major Four Herbs; Major Six Herbs; Stephania and Astragalus; Tang Gui and Ginseng Eight; Tang Gui and Indigo.
Cautions in Use: Do not use where there is Yin deficiency with Heat and thirst.

24. Auranti Fructus
枳殼

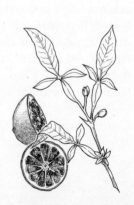

Latin Plant Name: Aurantii or Citri seu Ponciri
Pinyin Mandarin Name: *Zhi Ke*
Common English Name: Bitter Orange
Part of Plant Used: Dried fruit after seeds have been removed
Nature: Mildly cold
Taste: Bitter, sour

Meridians Entered: Spleen, Stomach
Common Usages: Most often used in formulas to treat symptoms of bloating and constipation due to food stagnation and indigestion; sometimes used for a stuffy sensation in the chest with yellow thick phlegm; also used for prolapse of the uterus, rectum, or stomach.
Traditional Usages and Functions: Disperses stagnated flow of vital Qi energy.
Common Formulas Used In: Bupleurum, Inula, and Cyperus.
Cautions in Use: Use with caution if there is little or no Spleen or Stomach function.

25. Auranti Immaturus
枳實

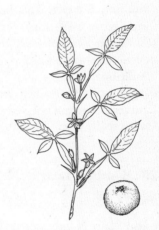

Latin Plant Name: Aurantii Immaturus or Fructus Citri seu Ponciri Immaturus
Pinyin Mandarin Name: *Zhi Shi*
Common English Name: Immature Fruit of Bitter Orange
Part of Plant Used: Dried fruit after seeds are removed
Nature: Mildly cold
Taste: Bitter, sour
Meridians Entered: Spleen, Stomach
Common Usages: This herb is most often used for its effect on symptoms of bloating *(OM: stomach accumulations)*, and may also be used to treat Organ prolapse and some cases of shock.
Traditional Usages and Functions: Breaks up stagnant Qi and reduces Accumulations; directs Qi downward and moves stool.
Common Formulas Used In: Apricot Seed and Linum.
Cautions in Use: Do not use where there is Qi deficiency or where there is a cold-deficient Stomach.

26. Avicularis

萹蓄

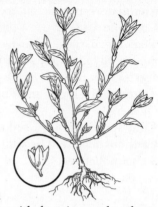

Latin Plant Name: Polygoni Avicularis
Pinyin Mandarin Name: *Bian Xu*
Common English Name: Avicularis or
Polygonum
Part of Plant Used: Whole plant
Nature: Mildly cold
Taste: Bitter
Meridians Entered: Bladder
Common Usages: This herb is used in
formulas to treat urinary-tract infections with burning and redness
(OM: damp heat conditions); also used internally and topically for parasite
infections in the colon and on the skin.
Traditional Usages and Functions: Promotes urination and clears
damp heat in the Bladder; expels parasites and stops itching.
Common Formulas Used In: Dianthus.
Cautions in Use: Use with caution if there is no damp heat.

27. Bamboo Leaf

淡竹葉

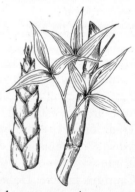

Latin Plant Name: Lophatheri Gracilis
Pinyin Mandarin Name: *Dan Zhu Ye*
Common English Name: Bamboo Leaf
Part of Plant Used: Stem and leaves
Nature: Cold
Taste: Sweet, bland
Meridians Entered: Heart, Stomach,
Bladder, Small Intestine
Common Usages: This herb is used in formulas to treat urinary-tract
infections with burning and redness *(OM: damp heat)*, especially where
there are symptoms of mouth and tongue sores with hot, swollen gums
(OM: heat in Stomach and Heart channels); also used with symptoms of
bronchitis, expectoraton of blood, insomnia, or convulsions.
Traditional Usages and Functions: Clears heat and lessens irritability; promotes urination and clears damp heat; releases exterior and disperses wind heat.

Common Formulas Used In: Lonicera and Forsythia.
Cautions in Use: Use with caution during pregnancy.

28. Biota
柏子仁

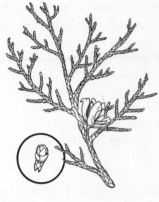

Latin Plant Name: Biotae Orientalis
Pinyin Mandarin Name: *Bai Zi Ren*
Common English Name: Arbor Vitae
Seeds
Part of Plant Used: Seed
Nature: Neutral
Taste: Sweet, acrid
Meridians Entered: Heart, Liver,
Spleen, Large Intestine
Common Usages: This herb is used in formulas to treat nervous disorders, elimination difficulties, and night sweats *(OM: deficient Yin).*
Traditional Usages and Functions: Nourishes the Heart and calms the Spirit; moistens Intestines.
Common Formulas Used In: Cerebral Tonic Pills; Ginseng and Zizyphus.
Cautions in Use: Use with caution where there are loose stools, dampness or phlegm imbalances.

29. Bupleurum
柴胡

Latin Plant Name: Bupleuri Radix
Pinyin Mandarin Name: *Chai Hu*
Common English Name: Bupleurum
Part of Plant Used: Whole plant
Nature: Cool
Taste: Bitter, slightly acrid
Meridians Entered: Liver, Gallbladder,
Pericardium
Common Usages: This herb is used in formulas to treat colds with chest congestion and alternating chills and fevers and other respiratory illnesses that

are at a superficial level in the body; also used to treat many imbalances of the Liver and Gallbladder, including hepatitis and cirrhosis; and to strengthen digestive and metabolic functions *(OM: internal heat, Liver fire, Spleen deficiency, and stagnant Liver Qi)*.

Traditional Usages and Functions: Resolves lesser Yang heat patterns; relaxes constrained Liver Qi; raises Yang Qi in cases of Spleen or Stomach Deficiency.

Common Formulas Used In: Bupleurum and Dragon Bone; Bupleurum, Inula, and Cyperus; Bupleurum and Tang Gui; Cimicafuga; Ginseng and Astragalus; Minor Bupleurum; Rehmannia and Magnetitum; Rhubarb and Scutellaria.

Cautions in Use: Do not use if there is a deficient-Yin cough or symptoms of Liver fire rising.

30. Burdock Fructus

牛蒡子

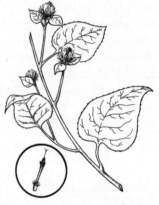

Latin Plant Name: Arctii Lappae
Pinyin Mandarin Name: *Niu Bang Zi*
Common English Name: Burdock Fruit
Part of Plant Used: Fruit
Nature: Slightly cold
Taste: Acrid, slightly bitter
Meridians Entered: Lungs, Stomach
Common Usages: This herb is used in formulas to treat symptoms of red and swollen throat, cough with yellow phlegm, fever, and measles; also used for other heat-related rashes and for carbuncles *(OM: imbalances of internal heat, wind heat, and wind dampness)*.

Traditional Usages and Functions: Disperses wind heat and benefits the throat; detoxifies fire poison; encourages rashes to surface; moistens Intestines.

Common Formulas Used In: Lonicera and Forsythia.

Cautions in Use: Do not use this herb when there are open sores or carbuncles, or where there is deficient Qi and diarrhea.

31. Capillaris

茵陳蒿

Latin Plant Name: Artemesia Capillaris
Pinyin Mandarin Name: *Yin Chen Hao*
Common English Name: Capillaris
Part of Plant Used: Young shoots and
leaves
Nature: Cool
Taste: Bitter, acrid
Meridians Entered: Spleen, Stomach,
Liver, Gallbladder
Common Usages: Formulas use this herb
most often for its effect in treating any kind of jaundice with accompanying eye and skin discoloration and dark urine *(OM: damp heat; Liver imbalance);* and to treat pain on the side and under ribs with accompanying nausea and appetite loss *(OM: Liver or Gallbladder imbalance).*
Traditional Usages and Functions: Clears damp heat from the Liver and Gallbladder and relieves jaundice; clears heat and relieves exterior conditions.
Common Formulas Used In: Rhubarb and Scutellaria.
Remarks: In cases of jaundice, see a practitioner immediately. This herb is combined with different types of herbs for different types of jaundice.
Cautions in Use: None.

32. Cardamom Seed

砂仁

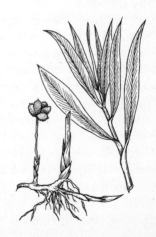

Latin Plant Name: Amomi Fructus seu
Semen
Pinyin Mandarin Name: *Sha Ren*
Common English Name: Cardamom
Seed
Part of Plant Used: Fruit
Nature: Warm
Taste: Acrid, aromatic
Meridians Entered: Spleen, Stomach,
Kidneys

Common Usages: This herb is used in formulas to treat stomach disorders, including stagnant or obstructed food in the stomach *(OM: stagnant Qi; dampness obstruction);* vomiting and diarrhea *(OM: internal cold and damp);* and to reduce uterine contractions in the event of threatened miscarriage.

Traditional Usages and Functions: Moves Qi and strengthens Stomach; promotes movement of food; transforms dampness and stops vomiting; calms the fetus.

Common Formulas Used In: Bupleurum, Inula, and Cyperus; Ginseng and Atractylodes; Hoelen and Polyporus.

Remarks: Because of cardamom's effectiveness in moving food through the digestive tract, it is used in formulas that have a strong tonic action to balance those formulas' tendencies to be damp in nature, a factor that may lead to stagnation.

Cardamom is added last when preparing raw herbs for drinking, since its aromatic qualities dissipate with long boiling.

Cautions in Use: Do not use this herb when there is a strong Yin deficiency or heat signs caused by Yin deficiency.

33. Cardamom Seed (infertile)

白豆蔻

Latin Plant Name: Amomi Cardamomi
Pinyin Mandarin Name: *Bai Dou Kou*
Common English Name: Cardamom
Seed (infertile)
Part of Plant Used: Fruit
Nature: Warm
Taste: Acrid, aromatic
Meridians Entered: Spleen, Stomach, Lung
Common Usages: This herb is used in formulas that treat abdominal bloating and poor digestion *(OM: dampness, stagnant Qi, or rebellious Qi),* and for nausea *(OM: internal cold and damp).*
Traditional Usages and Functions: Transforms dampness; warms Middle Burner and causes rebellious Qi to descend; moves Qi and transforms Stagnation; warms Lungs and Stomach.
Common Formulas Used In: Bupleurum, Inula, and Cyperus.
Remarks: Cardamom is added last when preparing raw herbs for drinking, since its aromatic qualities dissipate with long boiling.

Cautions in Use: Do not use this herb when there is a strong Yin or Blood deficiency. Use with caution when there are no signs of cold and damp in the Spleen and Stomach.

34. Carthamus Flower

紅花

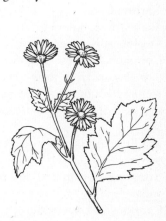

Latin Plant Name: Carthami Tinctorii
Pinyin Mandarin Name: *Hong Hua*
Common English Name: Safflower
Part of Plant Used: Flower
Nature: Warm
Taste: Acrid
Meridians Entered: Heart, Liver
Common Usages: This herb is used in formulas to treat menstrual imbalances and pain, lack of menstrual blood flow, postbirth abdominal pain, and traumatic injuries *(OM: stagnant and congealed Blood).*
Traditional Usages and Functions: Invigorates Blood and promotes menstruation; dispels Congealed Blood and alleviates pain; harmonizes Blood.
Common Formulas Used In: Pseudoginseng and Dragon Blood.
Cautions in Use: Do not use during pregnancy.

35. Chrysanthemum

菊花

Latin Plant Name: Chrysanthemi Morifolii
Pinyin Mandarin Name: *Ju Hua*
Common English Name: Chrysanthemum
Part of Plant Used: Flower head
Nature: Slightly cold
Taste: Sweet, slightly bitter
Meridians Entered: Lungs, Liver
Common Usages: This herb is used in formulas that treat rapid-onset

inflammatory conditions involving headache, fever, and red and painful tearing or dry eyes *(OM: wind-heat injuries; internal wind heat in Liver channel)*; also used to treat certain types of high blood pressure.

Traditional Usages and Functions: Disperses wind and clears heat; clears Liver and brightens the eyes; pacifies Liver and extinguishes wind; neutralizes toxins.

Common Formulas Used In: Prunella and Scutellaria; Rehmannia and Dogwood Fruit.

Remarks: The two types of flowers—white and yellow—have slightly different properties: the white flower is used more to nourish the Liver and clear the eyes; the yellow flower is used more for wind-heat symptoms. The flowers can be simmered a few minutes, cooled, and placed on the eyes to relieve pain and redness.

Cautions in Use: Do not use this herb when there is deficient Qi, poor appetite, or diarrhea.

36. Chrysanthemum (wild)

野菊花

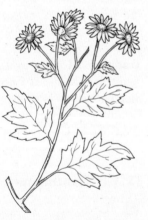

Latin Plant Name: Chrysanthemi Indici
Pinyin Mandarin Name: *Ye Ju Hua*
Common English Name:
Chrysanthemum (wild)
Part of Plant Used: Flower
Nature: Cool
Taste: Acrid, bitter
Meridians Entered: Lung, Liver
Common Usages: This herb is used in formulas to treat toxic skin imbalances such as boils or sores *(OM: fire poison)* and eczema *(OM: internal heat)*; also used in formulas to treat high blood pressure *(OM: related to Liver heat)*.

Traditional Usages and Functions: Quells fire and detoxifies fire poison.

Common Formulas Used In: Ilex and Evodia; Xanthium and Magnolia.

Cautions in Use: None.

37. Cimicifuga

升麻

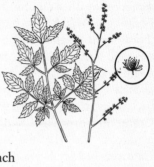

Latin Plant Name: Cimicifugae
Pinyin Mandarin Name: *Sheng Ma*
Common English Name: Black Cohosh
Part of Plant Used: Root
Nature: Cool
Taste: Sweet, acrid, slightly bitter
Meridians Entered: Lung, Spleen, Stomach
Common Usages: This herb is used in formulas that promote erup-
tion of the rash in measles and shorten the period of discomfort asso-
ciated with the disease *(OM: internal heat; deficient-Yang Qi);* also used
to treat other symptoms similar to those associated with measles,
including headache, fever, sore throat *(OM: exterior wind heat);*
and sores and ulcerations in the throat and mouth *(OM: Stomach fire
poison).*
Traditional Usages and Functions: Releases exterior and encourages
the rash of measles to surface; raises Yang Qi; detoxifies fire poison
affecting Stomach.
Common Formulas Used In: Cimicafuga; Ginseng and Astragalus.
Cautions in Use: Do not use this herb when there is an excess condition in the Upper Burner and a deficiency in the Lower Burner.

38. Cinnamon Bark

肉桂

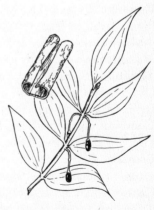

Latin Plant Name: Cinnamomi Cassiae
Pinyin Mandarin Name: *Rou Gui*
Common English Name: Cinnamon
Bark
Part of Plant Used: Bark
Nature: Hot
Taste: Acrid, sweet
Meridians Entered: Kidneys, Spleen,
Liver, Bladder
Common Usages: This herb is used in
formulas to treat chronic diarrhea with cold hands and feet *(OM: inter-
nal core coldness; deficient Kidney and Spleen Yang; deficient Qi and Blood),*

sometimes with symptoms of flushing of face and head, wheezing, and sweating *(OM: false heat symptoms in upper part of body).*

Traditional Usages and Functions: Promotes Yang growth in Kidneys and brings True Yang into system via Kidneys; warms Kidneys and fortifies Yang; warms the Middle Burner and disperses cold; warms the channels, promotes menstruation, and alleviates pain; leads the fire back to its source; generates Qi and Blood.

Common Formulas Used In: Ginseng and Tang Gui Ten; Rehmannia Eight; Tian Man and Eucommia; Tu-Huo and Loranthus.

Cautions in Use: Do not use during pregnancy. Do not use when there is a strong Yin deficiency or there are heat signs.

39. Cinnamon Twig

桂枝

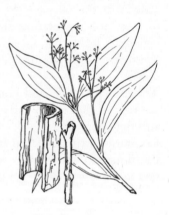

Latin Plant Name: Cinnamomi Cassiae
Pinyin Mandarin Name: *Gui Zhi*
Common English Name: Cinnamon Twig
Part of Plant Used: Twig
Nature: Warm
Taste: Acrid, sweet
Meridians Entered: Heart, Lungs, Bladder

Common Usages: This herb is used in formulas that promote sweating to treat exterior symptoms such as fever without sweating and weakness; also used for arthritic conditions, especially of the shoulders, and to remove edema by increasing circulation.

Traditional Usages and Functions: Adjusts Nutritive and Protective Qi levels; warms channels and disperses cold; moves Yang and transforms Qi; strengthens Heart Yang.

Common Formulas Used In: Bupleurum and Dragon Bone; Hoelen Five; Ma Huang; Pueraria Combination.

Remarks: Cinnamon twig is used in many formulas for its warm/sweet nature to enhance their warming and tonifying effects.

Cautions in Use: Use cautiously during pregnancy. Do not use this herb when there is a strong Yin deficiency, heat signs caused by Yin deficiency, or heat in the Blood with vomiting.

40. Cistanches

肉苁蓉

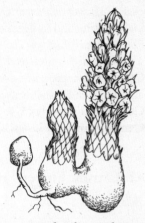

Latin Plant Name: Cistanches
Pinyin Mandarin Name: *Rou Cong Rong*
Common English Name: Cistanches
Part of Plant Used: Whole plant
Nature: Warm
Taste: Sweet, sour, salty
Meridians Entered: Kidneys, Large Intestine
Common Usages: This herb is used in formulas to treat symptoms of weak and cold lower back and knees along with impotence or infertility and general chilliness *(OM: promotes Kidney yang)*; also used to treat chronic constipation *(OM: with chronic deficiency of Qi and Blood)*.
Traditional Usages and Functions: Tonifies Kidneys and strengthens Yang; warms the Womb; moistens Intestines and facilitates passage of stool.
Common Formulas Used In: Cerebral Tonic Pills.
Cautions in Use: Do not use this herb when there is a strong Yin deficiency, heat signs, or diarrhea with symptoms of a weak Stomach and Spleen.

41. Citri Immaturi

青皮

Latin Plant Name: Citri Reticulatae Viride
Pinyin Mandarin Name: *Qing Pi*
Common English Name: Immature Tangerine (peel)
Part of Plant Used: Immature (green) fruit
Nature: Slightly warm
Taste: Acrid, bitter
Meridians Entered: Stomach, Liver, Gallbladder
Common Usages: This herb is used in formulas to treat pain and masses in abdomen with possible sensation of hernia, or pain in chest or

ribs *(OM: stagnant Liver Qi and excess phlegm);* also used to treat abdominal bloating and indigestion *(OM: stagnant digestive function. Do not confuse with poor digestion due to deficiency and weakness).*

Traditional Usages and Functions: Expedites the free flow of Liver Qi and alleviates pain; breaks up and reduces Qi accumulations; dries dampness and transforms phlegm.

Common Formulas Used In: Bupleurum, Inula, and Cyperus.

Cautions in Use: Use with caution where there is deficient Spleen Qi.

42. Citron, Finger Fructus

佛手

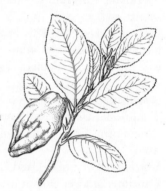

Latin Plant Name: Fructus Citri Sarcodactylis
Pinyin Mandarin Name: *Fou Shou*
Common English Name: Finger Citron Fruit
Part of Plant Used: Fruit
Nature: Slightly warm
Taste: Acrid, sour, bitter
Meridians Entered: Liver, Stomach, Spleen, Lungs

Common Usages: This herb is used in formulas to treat symptoms of vomiting, belching, poor appetite, or rib pain *(OM: stagnant Liver, Stomach, and Spleen Qi);* also used to strengthen digestive function and metabolism, and reduce phlegm in lungs and digestive system *(OM: poor circulation of Lung Qi; stagnation).*

Traditional Usages and Functions: Moves Qi and alleviates pain; harmonizes Stomach and strengthens Spleen; regulates circulation of Lung Qi and disperses phlegm.

Common Formulas Used In: Bupleurum, Inula, and Cyperus.

Cautions in Use: Use cautiously where there is no stagnant Qi, or if there is deficient Yin with excess heat signs.

43. Citrus Peel (aged)

陳皮

Latin Plant Name: Citri Reticulatae
Pinyin Mandarin Name: *Chen Pi*
Common English Name: Tangerine
Peel
Part of Plant Used: Fruit peel
Nature: Warm
Taste: Acrid, bitter, aromatic
Meridians Entered: Spleen, Stomach,
Lungs

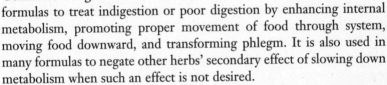

Common Usages: This herb is used in
formulas to treat indigestion or poor digestion by enhancing internal
metabolism, promoting proper movement of food through system,
moving food downward, and transforming phlegm. It is also used in
many formulas to negate other herbs' secondary effect of slowing down
metabolism when such an effect is not desired.

Traditional Usages and Functions: Moves Qi and strengthens
Spleen; dries dampness and transforms phlegm; directs Qi downward
and stops vomiting; helps prevent stagnation.

Common Formulas Used In: Agastache; Bupleurum, Inula, and
Cyperus; Citrus and Pinellia; Clematis and Stephania; Fritallaria
Extract Tablet; Ginseng and Astragaluls; Major Six Herbs.

Cautions in Use: Do not use this herb where there is a dry cough from
deficient Yin or Qi. Use cautiously where there are heat signs such as
expectoration of phlegm, or where there is thick yellow or green
phlegm with coughing.

44. Codonopsis

Latin Plant Name: Codonopsis Pilosulae
Pinyin Mandarin Name: *Dang Shen*
Common English Name: Codonopsis
Part of Plant Used: Root
Nature: Neutral
Taste: Sweet
Meridians Entered: Spleen, Lungs
Common Usages: This herb is used in formulas to treat fatigue with poor appetite where there is poor internal metabolism *(OM: stimulates function of Spleen and Stomach to normalize movement of fluids; tonifies Spleen and Lungs to metabolize and disperse Qi);* also used for chronic diarrhea *(OM: chronic Spleen Qi deficiency);* and to treat symptoms of easy bruising and prolapse of Organs and tissues such as uterus and hemorrhoids.
Traditional Usages and Functions: Tonifies Middle Burner and benefits Qi; tonifies Lungs; strengthens and tonifies Qi and nourishes fluids; builds Blood.
Common Formulas Used In: Tang Gui and Indigo.
Remarks: Codonopsis is often substituted for ginseng, although it is not as strong. Some practitioners consider codonopsis to be more damp than ginseng, thus requiring more care in use, especially with a serious collapse of Qi and Yang, a condition where ginseng shines as a treatment.
Cautions in Use: None.

45. Coix

薏苡仁

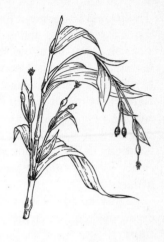

Latin Plant Name: Coicis Lachryma-Jobi
Pinyin Mandarin Name: *Yi Yi Ren*
Common English Name: Job's Tears (seed)
Part of Plant Used: Seed with the husk removed
Nature: Cool
Taste: Sweet, bland
Meridians Entered: Spleen, Stomach, Lungs, Large Intestine
Common Usages: This herb is used in formulas that promote urination; treat edema and arthritislike pain and spasms in the legs; reduce diarrhea; and assist digestion (*OM: internal dampness; deficient Spleen function; damp-heat conditions*).
Traditional Usages and Functions: Promotes urination and leaches out dampness; strengthens Spleen and stops diarrhea; clears heat and expels pus; expels wind dampness; clears damp heat.
Common Formulas Used In: Ginseng and Atractylodes.
Cautions in Use: Do not use during pregnancy.

46. Coptis

黄連

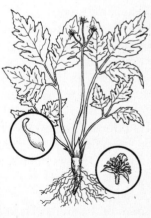

Latin Plant Name: Coptidis
Pinyin Mandarin Name: *Huang Lian*
Common English Name: Coptis
Part of Plant Used: Root
Nature: Cold
Taste: Bitter
Meridians Entered: Heart, Liver, Stomach, Large Intestine
Common Usages: This herb is used in formulas to treat many excess heat-related conditions including severe sore throats, high fevers, delirium, nosebleeds, and blood in stool, phlegm, or vomit (*OM: excess heat symptoms*).

Traditional Usages and Functions: Quells fire and detoxifies fire poison; clears heat and drains dampness; clears Heart fire; clears heat and stops bleeding; drains Stomach fire; clears heat topically.

Common Formulas Used In: Hoelen and Polyporus; Leonuris and Achyranthes; Tang Gui and Gardenia.

Remarks: Coptis is one of the stronger herbs with heat-clearing action and can be used for almost any excessive heat symptom. With severe symptoms, it is always best to consult a practitioner.

Cautions in Use: Do not use this herb when there is a strong Yin deficiency or cold-deficient Stomach, or diarrhea from deficient Spleen or Kidneys.

Coptis should not be used for long periods of time due to its cold and drying qualities, which may create deficient Spleen and Stomach imbalances.

47. Cornu Cervi

鹿茸

Latin Plant Name: Cornu Cervi Parvum
Pinyin Mandarin Name: *Lu Rong*
Common English Name: Velvet of Young Deer Horn
Part of Plant Used: Velvet of the horn
Nature: Warm
Taste: Sweet, salty
Meridians Entered: Liver, Kidneys
Common Usages: This herb is used in formulas to treat anemia after chronic disease, impotence, and weakness of back and knees with cold intolerance; also used to treat children for failure to thrive, mental retardation, learning disabilities, and skeletal deformities (*OM: deficient Yang, deficient Blood, and deficient Kidney Yang; deficient Essence).*

Traditional Usages and Functions: Tonifies Kidneys and fortifies Yang; tonifies the Governing Channel, benefits Essence and Blood, and strengthens sinews and bones; bolsters the Penetrating and Conception Channels and strengthens the Girdle Channel; tonifies and nourishes Qi and Blood.

Common Formulas Used In: Tian Qi and Eucommia.

Cautions in Use: Do not use this herb when there is a strong Yin deficiency or heat signs caused by Yin deficiency.

48. Cornus

山茱萸

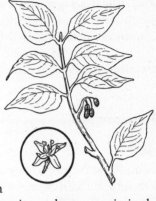

Latin Plant Name: Corni Officinalis
Pinyin Mandarin Name: *Shan Zhu Yu*
Common English Name: Cornus
Part of Plant Used: Root
Nature: Slightly warm
Taste: Sour
Meridians Entered: Kidneys, Lungs, Liver
Common Usages: This herb is used in formulas to treat copious sweating, leaking urine and sperm, pain in the lower back and knees, dizziness, poor hearing, ringing in the ears, prolonged menstruation, and in extreme cases, shock *(OM: "leaking" Essence)*.
Traditional Usages and Functions: Stabilizes Kidneys and Liver, and contains Essence; stabilizes menses and stops bleeding; stops excessive sweating and supports that which has collapsed.
Common Formulas Used In: Anemarrhena, Phellodendron, and Rehmannia; Eight Immortal Long Life Pill; Rehmannia and Dogwood Fruit; Rehmannia and Magnetitum; Rehmannia Eight; Rehmannia Six.
Cautions in Use: Do not use this herb when there is painful or difficult urination, or if there are heat and dampness symptoms.

49. Corydalis

延胡索

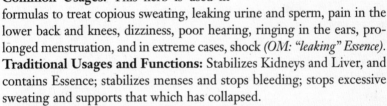

Latin Plant Name: Corydalis Ambigua
Pinyin Mandarin Name: *Yan Hu Suo*
Common English Name: Corydalis
Part of Plant Used: Root
Nature: Warm
Taste: Acrid, bitter
Meridians Entered: Liver, Spleen, Stomach, Lungs
Common Usages: This herb is used both in formulas and singly to relieve pain *(OM: congealed Blood and stagnant Qi)*; also used for insomnia and lower-back pain.

Traditional Usages and Functions: Invigorates Blood and alleviates pain; moves Qi and alleviates pain.

Common Formulas Used In: Bupleurum, Inula, and Cyperus; Corydalis; Corydalis Tuber; Tang Gui and Indigo.

Cautions in Use: Do not use during pregnancy.

50. Curcuma

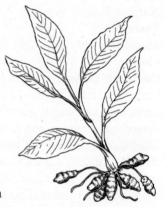

Latin Plant Name: Curcumae
Pinyin Mandarin Name: *Jiang Huang*
Common English Name: Turmeric
Part of Plant Used: Root
Nature: Warm
Taste: Acrid, bitter
Meridians Entered: Spleen, Stomach, Liver
Common Usages: This herb is used in formulas to relieve pain, including arthritic or traumatic pain, abdominal pain, and menstrual pain (*OM: Blood or Qi stasis*).

Traditional Usages and Functions: Invigorates Blood and promotes menstruation; moves Qi and alleviates pain; expels wind and moves Blood.

Common Formulas Used In: Bupleurum, Inula, and Cyperus; Qiang-Huo and Turmeric.

Cautions in Use: Do not use during pregnancy. Do not use where there is deficient Blood with no signs of stagnant Qi or congealed Blood.

51. Cuscuta

菟絲子

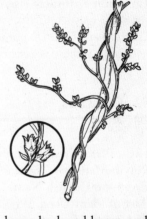

Latin Plant Name: Cuscutae
Pinyin Mandarin Name: *Tu Si Zi*
Common English Name: Cuscuta
Part of Plant Used: Seeds
Nature: Neutral
Taste: Acrid, sweet
Meridians Entered: Liver, Kidneys
Common Usages: This herb is used in formulas to treat impotence, nighttime sperm leakage, premature ejaculation, ringing in the ears, frequent urination, sore lower back and knees, and leukorrhea *(OM: deficient Kidney Qi and deficient Essence);* also used for blurred vision, dry eyes, and eyes that tire easily.

Traditional Usages and Functions: Tonifies Kidneys and benefits Essence; calms the fetus; benefits Spleen and Kidneys and stops diarrhea; tonifies Liver and brightens eyes.

Common Formulas Used In: Concha Marguerita and Ligustrum.

Cautions in Use: None.

52. Cyperus

香附

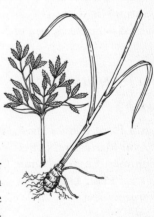

Latin Plant Name: Cyperi Rotundi
Pinyin Mandarin Name: *Xiang Fu*
Common English Name: Cyperus
Part of Plant Used: Root
Nature: Slightly Warm
Taste: Acrid, slightly bitter, sweet
Meridians Entered: Liver, Triple Burner
Common Usages: This herb is used in formulas that relieve pain, particularly the pain of menstruation *(OM: deficient/stagnant Qi and Liver Qi)*, without a "numbing" effect.

Traditional Usages and Functions: Circulates Qi and resolves constrained Liver Qi; regulates menstruation and alleviates pain.

Common Formulas Used In: Bupleurum, Inula, and Cyperus; Cyperus and Ligusticum.

Cautions in Use: Do not use where there is deficient Qi without stagnation, or if there is deficient Yin with heat.

53. Dianthus

瞿麥

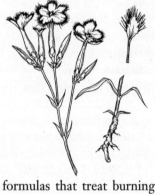

Latin Plant Name: Dianthi
Pinyin Mandarin Name: *Qu Mai*
Common English Name: Dianthus
Part of Plant Used: Whole plant
Nature: Cold
Taste: Bitter
Meridians Entered: Heart, Kidneys, Small Intestine, Bladder

Common Usages: This herb is used in formulas that treat burning urine, irregular menstruation, and constipation *(OM: damp Heat conditions)*.

Traditional Usages and Functions: Clears heat and promotes urination; breaks up congealed Blood; promotes movement of stool.

Common Formulas Used In: Dianthus.

Cautions in Use: Do not use during pregnancy. Do not use where there is deficient Spleen or Kidneys.

54. Dioscoria

山藥

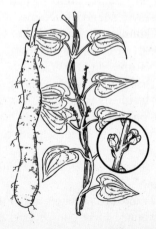

Latin Plant Name: Dioscoria Oppositae
Pinyin Mandarin Name: *Shan Yao*
Common English Name: Chinese Yam
Part of Plant Used: Root
Nature: Neutral
Taste: Sweet
Meridians Entered: Kidney, Lung, Spleen

Common Usages: This neutral herb is used in formulas as a tonic to treat most symptoms of chronic weakness, including chronic diarrhea, fatigue, leukorrhea, sperm leakage, spontaneous sweating, poor appetite, and asthma with dry cough; also can be applied locally for skin eruptions.

Traditional Usages and Functions: Tonifies and benefits Spleen and Stomach; benefits Lungs and nourishes Kidneys; nourishes base of body through digestive stabilization.

Common Formulas Used In: Anemarrhena, Phellodendron, and Rehmannia; Eight Immortal Long Life Pill; Ginseng and Atractylodes; Rehmannia and Dogwood Fruit; Rehmannia and Magnetitum; Rehmannia Eight; Rehmannia Six.

Cautions in Use: Do not use where there is a strong excess condition with dampness.

55. Dipsacus

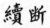

Latin Plant Name: Dipsaci
Pinyin Mandarin Name: *Xu Duan*
Common English Name: Dipsacus
Part of Plant Used: Root
Nature: Slightly warm
Taste: Bitter, acrid
Meridians Entered: Liver, Kidney
Common Usages: Dipsacus is renowned for its healing effects in treating fractures and other injuries, and may be used both internally and externally for those condi-

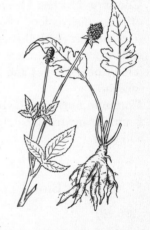

tions. It is also used in formulas to treat soreness of the lower back and legs due to weakness, and to treat complications of pregnancy that also are due to weakness, including bleeding and threatened miscarriage.

Traditional Usages and Functions: Tonifies Liver and Kidneys and strengthens sinews and bones; promotes circulation of Blood; stops uterine bleeding and calms the fetus.

Common Formulas Used In: Tang Gui and Indigo.

Cautions in Use: Do not use this herb where there is deficient Yin or strong signs of heat.

56. Dolichos

白扁豆

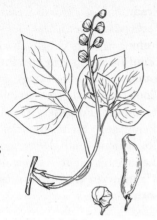

Latin Plant Name: Dolichoris Lablab
Pinyin Mandarin Name: *Bian Dou* or *Bai Bian Dou*
Common English Name: Hyacinth Bean
Part of Plant Used: Whole bean is used; and sometimes the bean, leaf, root, and flower
Nature: Neutral
Taste: Sweet
Meridians Entered: Spleen, Stomach
Common Usages: This herb is used in formulas to treat vomiting and diarrhea due to food poisoning or extreme heat exposure/sunstroke *(OM: summer heat);* also used to treat diarrhea *(OM: deficient Spleen)* and leukorrhea *(OM: deficient Spleen).*
Traditional Usages and Functions: Clears summer heat; strengthens Spleen.
Common Formulas Used In: Ginseng and Atractylodes.
Cautions in Use: Do not use this herb where there is alternating chills and fever.

57. Dragon Blood

血竭

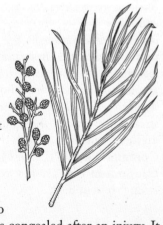

Latin Plant Name: Sanguis Draconis
Pinyin Mandarin Name: *Xue Jie*
Common English Name: Dragon's Blood
Part of Plant Used: Resin from the fruit and stem
Nature: Neutral
Taste: Sweet, salty
Meridians Entered: Heart, Liver
Common Usages: This herb is used to stop bleeding and to move blood that has congealed after an injury. It also has mild pain-relieving effects.

Traditional Usages and Functions: Dispels congealed Blood and alleviates pain; stops bleeding; protects surface of ulcer, prevents decay, and promotes healing.

Common Formulas Used In: Pseudoginseng and Dragon Blood.

Cautions in Use: Do not use this herb where there is deficient Yin /hot Blood. Use with caution where there are no symptoms of Blood stasis.

58. Dragon Bone

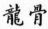 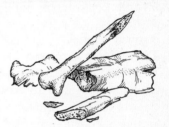

Latin Plant Name: Os Draconis
Pinyin Mandarin Name: *Long Gu*
Common English Name: Fossilized Bones
Part of Plant Used: Crushed fossilized bones
Nature: Neutral
Taste: Sweet, astringent
Meridians Entered: Heart, Liver, Kidneys
Common Usages: This herb is used in formulas to treat insomnia, anxiety, and emotional stress *(OM: weak or rebellious Spirit)*; blurred vision, dizziness, and poor temper *(rebellious Liver Qi)*; also used to treat leakage of sperm, excessive sweating, vaginal secretions, and bleeding *(OM: deficient or leaking Fluids)*.

Traditional Usages and Functions: Settles and calms the Spirit; pacifies Liver and restrains floating Yang; prevents leakage of fluids.

Common Formulas Used In: Bupleurum and Dragon Bone.

Cautions in Use: Do not use this herb where there are signs of an exterior excess hot or cold condition, or where there are heat and dampness symptoms.

59. Dragon Teeth

龍齒

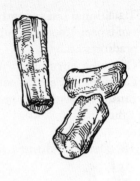

Latin Plant Name: Dens Draconis
Pinyin Mandarin Name: *Long Chi*
Common English Name: Fossilized Teeth
Part of Plant Used: Crushed fossilized teeth
Nature: Neutral
Taste: Sweet, astringent
Meridians Entered: Heart, Liver, Kidneys
Common Usages: This cooling and astringent herb is used to treat many of the same symptoms as Dragon Bone, but it is especially useful for treating dream-disturbed sleep or nightmares in children.
Traditional Usages and Functions: See Dragon Bone (No. 58).
Common Formulas Used In: Cerebral Tonic Pills.
Remarks: A rare and infrequently used mineral "herb" that has many of the same healing properties as Dragon Bone. Made by crushing the fossilized teeth of large mammals and reptiles.
Cautions in Use: Do not use this herb where there are signs of an exterior excess hot or cold condition, or where there are heat and dampness symptoms.

60. Eclipta

旱蓮草

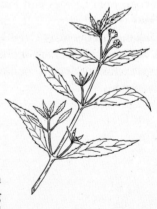

Latin Plant Name: Ecliptae Prostratae
Pinyin Mandarin Name: *Han Lian Cao*
Common English Name: Eclipta
Part of Plant Used: Whole plant
Nature: Cool
Taste: Sweet, sour
Meridians Entered: Liver, Kidneys
Common Usages: This herb is used in formulas to treat spontaneous bleeding from nose, uterus, and Lungs, and blood in urine *(OM: heat in Blood)*; also used to treat dizziness, blurred vision,

ringing in the ears, premature graying of hair, vertigo, loss of teeth, and sore back and knees *(OM: deficient Liver and Kidney Yin syndromes)*.

Traditional Usages and Functions: Nourishes and tonifies Liver and Kidney Yin; cools Blood and stops bleeding.

Common Formulas Used In: Concha Marguerita and Ligustrum.

Cautions in Use: Do not use where there is a deficiency cold pattern in the Liver or Kidneys.

61. Ephedra

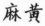

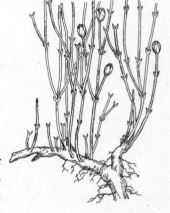

Latin Plant Name: Ephedra Sinensis
Pinyin Mandarin Name: *Ma Huang*
Common English Name: Ephedra
Part of Plant Used: Twigs and stems
Nature: Warm
Taste: Acrid, bitter
Meridians Entered: Lungs, Bladder
Common Usages: Ephedra is one of the major herbs used to treat wheezing *(OM: poor Lung Qi circulation)*. It is also used in formulas that induce sweating where there are symptoms of fever with no sweating, together with chills and headache *(OM: exterior cold)*; also used to treat asthma and allergies *(OM: wind-cold conditions)*.

Traditional Usages and Functions: Releases exterior and disperses cold; facilitates normal circulation of Lung Qi and controls wheezing; promotes urination and reduces edema.

Common Formulas Used In: Ma Huang; Pueraria Combination.

Remarks: Avoid using at night. Ephedra is a mild stimulant and may interfere with sleep, especially if the person already has insomnia.

Cautions in Use: Do not use this herb where there is high blood pressure or cardiac asthma. Use with caution in deficient conditions with chronic sweating or wheezing.

62. Eucommia Bark

杜仲

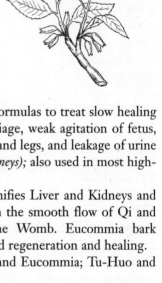

Latin Plant Name: Eucommiae
Ulmoidis
Pinyin Mandarin Name: *Du Zhong*
Common English Name: Eucommia
Bark
Part of Plant Used: Bark
Nature: Warm
Taste: Sweet, slightly acrid
Meridians Entered: Liver, Kidneys
Common Usages: This herb is used in formulas to treat slow healing
of tissues after injury, threatened miscarriage, weak agitation of fetus,
fatigue, weak, sore, or painful lower back and legs, and leakage of urine
and sperm *(OM: weakness in Liver and Kidneys);* also used in most high-
blood-pressure formulas.
Traditional Usages and Functions: Tonifies Liver and Kidneys and
strengthens the sinews and bones; aids in the smooth flow of Qi and
Blood; pacifies the fetus and calms the Womb. Eucommia bark
increases circulation to the tissues to speed regeneration and healing.
Common Formulas Used In: Tian Qi and Eucommia; Tu-Huo and
Loranthus.
Cautions in Use: Do not use this herb where there is a Yin deficiency
pattern with heat signs.

63. Evodia

吴茱萸

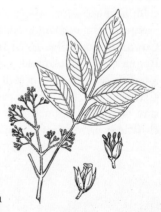

Latin Plant Name: Evodia Rutaecarpae
Pinyin Mandarin Name: *Wu Zhu Yu*
Common English Name: Evodia Fruit
Part of Plant Used: Fruit
Nature: Warm
Taste: Acrid, bitter, slightly toxic
Meridians Entered: Spleen, Stomach,
Liver, Kidneys
Common Usages: This herb is used in
formulas to treat vomiting due to phlegm

and cold conditions in the Stomach with symptoms of nausea, drooling clear or white fluid, headaches, decreased taste, and sensation of coldness or hernia pain in abdomen *(OM: interior cold and dampness)*; vomiting with sour vomitus and symptoms of flank pain *(OM: rebellious Stomach Qi; cold-damp leg Qi)*; and cold-related diarrhea *(Spleen and Stomach deficiency; interior cold dampness)*; also useful in expelling pinworms and tapeworms.

Traditional Usages and Functions: Disperses cold, alleviates pain, and stops vomiting; redirects rebellious Qi downward and stops vomiting; warms Spleen, stops diarrhea, and expels cold dampness.

Common Formulas Used In: Ilex and Evodia.

Cautions in Use: Do not use this herb where there is a Yin deficiency with heat signs.

64. Fennel
小茴香

Latin Plant Name: Foeniculi Vulgaris
Pinyin Mandarin Name: *Xiao Hui Xiang* or *Hui Xiang*
Common English Name: Fennel Fruit
Part of Plant Used: Fruit
Nature: Warm
Taste: Acrid
Meridians Entered: Spleen, Stomach, Liver, Kidneys
Common Usages: This herb is used in formulas that stimulate and warm digestive organs to aid digestive function *(OM: reduces stagnation)*; and to treat symptoms such as sensation of hernia or pain in testicles *(OM: cold in Liver and Middle Burner)*.

Traditional Usages and Functions: Regulates Qi and alleviates pain; warms Middle Burner and pacifies Stomach.

Common Formulas Used In: Tang Gui and Indigo.

Cautions in Use: Use carefully where there is Yin deficiency with heat signs.

65. Forsythia Fruit

連翹

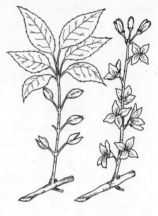

Latin Plant Name: Forsythia Suspensae
Pinyin Mandarin Name: *Lian Qiao*
Common English Name: Forsythia
Part of Plant Used: Fruit
Nature: Cool
Taste: Bitter, slightly acrid
Meridians Entered: Lungs, Heart, Liver, Gallbladder
Common Usages: This herb is used in formulas to treat symptoms of common cold where there is high fever, hot skin, lymphatic swelling (nodules), and/or urinary-tract infection (*OM: excess wind/hot/damp conditions*).
Traditional Usages and Functions: Clears heat and poison and dissipates nodules; expels externally contracted wind heat.
Common Formulas Used In: Lonicera and Forsythia; Xanthium and Magnolia.
Cautions in Use: Do not use this herb where there is deficient Spleen and Stomach diarrhea, or where there is fever with deficient Qi. Do not use where there are carbuncles that have already ulcerated, or if there are cold-type ulcers.

66. Frankincense Gum

乳香

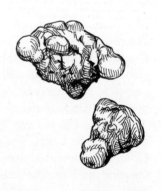

Latin Plant Name: Gummi Olibanum
Pinyin Mandarin Name: *Ru Xiang*
Common English Name: Frankincense Gum
Part of Plant Used: Gum resin
Nature: Warm
Taste: Acrid, warm
Meridians Entered: Heart, Liver, Spleen
Common Usages: Applied topically, this herb is used as an antiseptic and to reduce heat and swelling. Internally, it reduces swelling and helps with symptoms of pain associated with menstruation, early stages of carbuncles, sores, and swellings, and pain on the skin and in the

mouth *(OM: congealed Blood pain)*; also helps with trunk pain *(OM: due to congealed Blood)*, and spasm and rigidity *(OM: due to wind-damp obstruction)*.

Traditional Usages and Functions: Invigorates Blood and promotes circulation of Qi; relaxes sinews, activates channels, and alleviates pain; reduces swelling and promotes healing.

Common Formulas Used In: Pseudoginseng and Dragon Blood; Tian Qi and Eucommia.

Cautions in Use: Do not use during pregnancy.

67. Fritillaria

川貝母

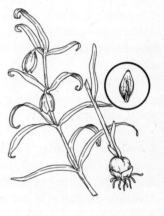

Latin Plant Name: Fritillariae Cirrhosae
Pinyin Mandarin Name: *Chuan Bei Mu*
Common English Name: Fritillaria
Part of Plant Used: Bulb
Nature: Cool
Taste: Sweet, bitter
Meridians Entered: Lungs, Heart
Common Usages: This herb is used in formulas that treat most any type of cough *(OM: except coughs associated with deficient Spleen)*, and various types of nodular formations *(OM: phlegm-fire hardening)*; also used to treat chronic bronchitis, tuberculosis, and chronic cough with sparse or hardened phlegm.

Traditional Usages and Functions: Clears heat, transforms phlegm, and stops coughing; clears heat and dissipates nodules.

Common Formulas Used In: Apricot Seed and Fritillaria; Fritillaria Extract Tablet.

Cautions in Use: Do not use where there is a deficient cold-phlegm pattern in the Spleen or Stomach.

68. Gardenia Fruit

栀子

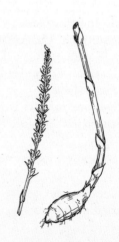

Latin Plant Name: Gardenia Jasminoidis
Pinyin Mandarin Name: *Zhi Zi*
Common English Name: Gardenia Fruit
Part of Plant Used: Fruit
Nature: Cold
Taste: Bitter
Meridians Entered: Liver, Lungs, Heart,
Gallbladder, Stomach, Triple Warmer
Common Usages: This herb is used in formulas to treat bladder infections, jaundice, ulcerations, spontaneous bleeding without trauma, and insomnia and irritability due to fever *(OM: heat or toxins in Blood)*.
Traditional Usages and Functions: Clears heat and alleviates irritability; drains damp heat in any of the three Burners; cools Blood and stops bleeding; reduces swelling and moves congealed Blood due to trauma.
Common Formulas Used In: Cyperus and Ligusticum; Dianthus; Gentiana; Tang Gui and Gardenia.
Remarks: May have a laxative effect.
Cautions in Use: Do not use this herb where there is cold-deficiency diarrhea.

69. Gastrodia

天麻

Latin Plant Name: Gastrodia Elatae
Pinyin Mandarin Name: *Tian Ma*
Common English Name: Gastrodia
Part of Plant Used: Root
Nature: Neutral
Taste: Sweet
Meridians Entered: Liver
Common Usages: This herb is used in formulas to treat spasms, convulsions, paralysis, numbness, cramping, and/or dizziness *(OM: Liver-wind imbalances and symptoms)*.

Traditional Usages and Functions: Pacifies Liver and extinguishes wind; extinguishes wind and alleviates pain; disperses painful obstructions.

Common Formulas Used In: Cerebral Tonic Pills; Leonuris and Achyranthes.

Remarks: Gastrodia is usually combined with other herbs to enhance their specific warming or cooling actions as appropriate to particular symptoms. Given the seriousness of many of these symptoms, consultation with a practitioner is recommended.

Cautions in Use: Use with caution where there are deficient-Yin symptoms.

70. Gelatinum Asini

阿膠

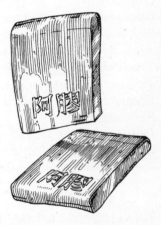

Latin Plant Name: Gelatinum Asini
Pinyin Mandarin Name: *E Jiao*
Common English Name: Gelatin from the skin of an Ass
Part of Plant Used: Prepared gelatin
Nature: Neutral
Taste: Sweet
Meridians Entered: Lungs, Liver, Kidneys
Common Usages: This herb is used to stop chronic bleeding and enhance recovery from excessive bleeding. It is most often used in formulas that treat anemia, tuberculosis, dry cough with bloody sputum, bleeding fibroids, and endometriosis; also used to raise blood platelet count, and to stop bleeding and spotting during pregnancy *(OM: builds Lung Yin and nourishes Blood)*.

Traditional Usages and Functions: Nourishes Blood; nourishes Blood and stops bleeding; nourishes Yin and moistens Lungs.

Common Formulas Used In: Leonuris and Achyranthes.

Remarks: Dissolve the gelatin in warm water before adding it to tea, or use alone after straining.

Cautions in Use: Do not use this herb where there is an exterior excess condition. Use with caution if there is deficent Spleen and/or Stomach.

71. Gentiana Macro

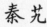

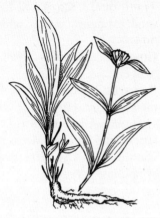

Latin Plant Name: Gentiana Macrophyllae
Pinyin Mandarin Name: *Qin Jiao*
Common English Name: Gentiana Macro
Part of Plant Used: Root
Nature: Neutral
Taste: Bitter, acrid
Meridians Entered: Liver, Stomach, Gallbladder
Common Usages: This herb is used in formulas to treat arthritis, jaundice, and chronic low-grade fevers, especially if there is constipation due to dryness (*OM: damp wind in joints; damp heat; deficient Yin*).
Traditional Usages and Functions: Expels wind dampness; removes deficient heat; removes jaundice; moistens Intestines and moves stool.
Common Formulas Used In: Clematis and Stephania; Tu-Huo and Eucommia.
Cautions in Use: Do not use this herb where there is frequent urination, chronic pain with consistent weight loss, or Spleen-deficiency diarrhea with a weak constitution.

72. Gentiana Scabra

龍胆草

Latin Plant Name: Gentianae Scabrae
Pinyin Mandarin Name: *Long Dan Cao*
Common English Name: Chinese Gentian
Part of Plant Used: Root
Nature: Cold
Taste: Bitter
Meridians Entered: Liver, Stomach, Gallbladder, Bladder
Common Usages: This herb is used in formulas to treat bloodshot eyes or conjunctivitis, bitter taste in mouth, high blood pressure, acute urinary infection, testicular and vaginal pain,

leukorrhea, swelling, fever, spasms, and/or ear imbalances *(OM: Lower Burner damp heat and fire in Liver or Gallbladder Channels)*.

Traditional Usages and Functions: Drains damp heat from Liver and Gallbladder Channels; drains and pacifies excessive Liver fire.

Common Formulas Used In: Gentiana.

Cautions in Use: Do not use this herb where there is a deficient Spleen and Stomach pattern with diarrhea, or where there is no true heat, dampness, or fire symptoms.

73. Ginger (fresh)

生薑

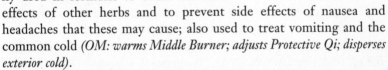

Latin Plant Name: Zingiberis Officinalis
Pinyin Mandarin Name: *Sheng Jiang*
Common English Name: Fresh Ginger
Part of Plant Used: Root
Nature: Hot
Taste: Acrid
Meridians Entered: Lungs, Stomach, Spleen
Common Usages: This herb is primarily used in formulas to offset the toxic effects of other herbs and to prevent side effects of nausea and headaches that these may cause; also used to treat vomiting and the common cold *(OM: warms Middle Burner; adjusts Protective Qi; disperses exterior cold)*.

Traditional Usages and Functions: Releases exterior and disperses cold; warms Middle Burner and alleviates vomiting; disperses cold and alleviates coughing; reduces poisonous effects of other herbs; adjusts Nutritive and Protective Qi.

Common Formulas Used In: Agastache; Bupleurum and Dragon Bone; Bupleurum and Tang Gui; Citrus and Pinellia; Clematis and Stephania; Ginseng and Astragalus; Ginseng and Longan; Major Six Herbs; Minor Bupleurum; Pueraria Combination; Qiang-Huo and Turmeric; Stephania and Astragalus.

Cautions in Use: Do not use this herb where there is a Lung heat pattern or summer heat with vomiting.

74. Gingko Biloba (kernel)

白果

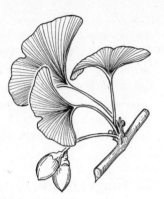

Latin Plant Name: Ginkgo Biloba
Pinyin Mandarin Name: *Ying Xing*
Common English Name: Ginkgo Nut
Part of Plant Used: Seed
Nature: Neutral
Taste: Sweet, bitter
Meridians Entered: Lungs, Kidneys
Common Usages: Gingko seeds are used
to treat chronic coughs, asthma, tubercu-
losis, bladder infections, frequent urination, and leukorrhea *(OM: defi-
cient Lung Qi; deficient Kidney yin; damp heat).*

Traditional Usages and Functions: Consolidates Lung Qi, strengthens Lungs, and relieves wheezing and coughing; expels phlegm;
astringes damp heat and stops discharges; stabilizes Lower Burner.

Common Formulas Used In: Gingko seeds are more properly considered a food and are used alone, raw or cooked, as a nutritional supplement. They are also used in capsule form as a supplement to
formulas that treat coughing and asthma, such as Ma Huang.

Gingko root is most often used to treat chronic cases of involuntary
ejaculation.

Gingko leaves, in capsule or tablet forms, are renowned for their
effectiveness in treating a wide variety of cerebral and circulatory problems, including migraine headaches, vertigo, memory dysfunction,
stroke, coronary thrombosis, and Alzheimer's disease.

Cautions in Use: Do not use where there are excess cold-damp symptoms. The kernels are mildly toxic and should not be taken either in
large quantities or over a long period of time. Use cautiously and in
small doses with children. (Consultation with a practitioner is recommended.) The root and leaves are not toxic.

75. Ginseng

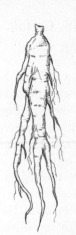

Latin Plant Name: Panax Ginseng
Pinyin Mandarin Name: *Ren Shen*
Common English Name: Ginseng
Part of Plant Used: Root
Nature: Slightly warm
Taste: Sweet, slightly bitter
Meridians Entered: Spleen, Lung, Heart
Common Usages: This herb is used in formulas to treat almost any kind of deficiency. Ginseng is renowned for tonifying Original Qi, which supplements all the other types of Qi. Ginseng has so many therapeutic uses that it is easier to list the few things for which is it is contraindicated (see "Cautions in Use" below).

Traditional Usages and Functions: Powerfully tonifies Original Qi; tonifies Lungs and benefits Qi; Strengthens Spleen and tonifies Stomach; benefits Yin and generates Fluids; benefits Heart Qi and calms Spirit.

Common Formulas Used In: Bupleurum and Dragon Bone; Ginseng and Astragalus; Ginseng and Atractylodes; Ginseng and Longan; Ginseng and Tang Gui Ten; Ginseng and Zizyphus; Major Four Herbs; Major Six Herbs; Minor Bupleurum; Panax Ginseng Capsules; Tang Gui and Ginseng Eight; Tian Man and Eucommia; Tu-Huo and Loranthus.

Remarks: If you are interested, there are numerous books about Ginseng. The bibliography at the end of this book lists several of them.

Cautions in Use: Do not use Ginseng where there is deficient Yin with heat signs, damp heat or excess heat patterns, or ascending Liver Yang. Do not use when high blood pressure is present, or if there are beginning symptoms of an exterior condition such as the common cold. Overuse of ginseng can lead to headache, insomnia, palpitations, or increased blood pressure.

76. Grifola

猪 苓

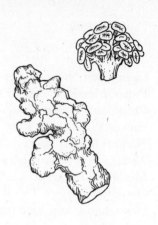

Latin Plant Name: Polypori Umbellati
Pinyin Mandarin Name: *Zhu Ling*
Common English Name: Grifola or Polyporus Fungus
Part of Plant Used: Central part of the fungus
Nature: Slightly cool
Taste: Sweet, bland
Meridians Entered: Spleen, Kidneys, Bladder
Common Usages: This herb is used in formulas to treat edema and associated symptoms of sparse urination and diarrhea *(OM: stagnant dampness)*.
Traditional Usages and Functions: Promotes urination and leaches out dampness.
Common Formulas Used In: Hoelen and Polyporus; Hoelen Five.
Cautions in Use: Do not use this herb where there is no dampness or for a prolonged period of time, because it may injure the Yin.

77. Haliotidis

石 决 明

Latin Plant Name: Concha Haliotidis
Pinyin Mandarin Name: *Shi Kue Ming*
Common English Name: Abalone Shell
Part of Plant Used: Whole shell
Nature: Slightly cold
Taste: Salty
Meridians Entered: Liver, Kidneys
Common Usages: This herb is used in formulas to treat high blood pressure, eye redness with light sensitivity, blurred vision, glaucoma, cataracts, headaches behind eyes, and spasms *(OM: Liver imbalances with heat symptoms)*.
Traditional Usages and Functions: Quells fire and causes Yang to descend; brightens eyes and causes superficial visual obstructions to recede.

Common Formulas Used In: Rehmannia and Dogwood Fruit.
Cautions in Use: Do not use during pregnancy. Not useful in most cases where there are no heat symptoms.

78. Inula

旋覆花

Latin Plant Name: Inula
Pinyin Mandarin Name: *Xuan Fu Hua*
Common English Name: Inula
Part of Plant Used: Flower
Nature: Slightly warm
Taste: Bitter, acrid
Meridians Entered: Lungs, Liver, Stomach, Spleen
Common Usages: This herb is used in formulas to treat symptoms of vomiting and belching, coughing and wheezing with large amounts of phlegm, or asthmatic bronchitis with large amounts of phlegm. *(OM: to treat "rebellious" Lung, Spleen, or Stomach functions, where these Organ functions are not operating in "normal" fashion).*
Traditional Usages and Functions: Redirects Qi downward and expels phlegm; stops vomiting and calms rebellion; provides mildly warming action.
Common Formulas Used In: Bupleurum, Inula, and Cyperus.
Cautions in Use: Do not use this herb where there is deficiency, or a cough that is due to wind and heat.

79. Isatidis

板蘭根

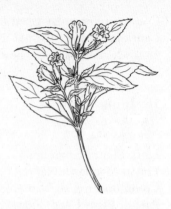

Latin Plant Name: Isatidis seu Baphica-canthi
Pinyin Mandarin Name: *Ban Lan Gen*
Common English Name: Isatidis
Part of Plant Used: Root
Nature: Cold
Taste: Bitter
Meridians Entered: Liver, Stomach, Lung
Common Usages: This herb is used in formulas to treat feverish flus; also used to treat symptoms of mumps, influenza, infectious hepatitis, and meningitis *(OM: heat in Blood)*.
Traditional Usages and Functions: Quells heat, detoxifies fire poison, and benefits the throat.
Common Formulas Used In: Ilex and Evodia.
Cautions in Use: Do not use this herb when the person is weak or if there is no fire poison.

80. Juncus

燈芯草

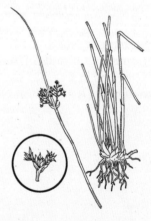

Latin Plant Name: Junci Effusi
Pinyin Mandarin Name: *Deng Xin Cao*
Common English Name: Juncus
Part of Plant Used: Pith
Nature: Slightly cold
Taste: Sweet, bland
Meridians Entered: Heart, Lungs, Small Intestine
Common Usages: This herb is used in formulas to treat Bladder and urinary-tract infections, particularly those created by "heat" conditions where there is concentrated urine and sometimes insomnia and mental disturbances, especially in children, with symptoms worsening at night. *(OM: damp heat; heat in Heart)*.
Traditional Usages and Functions: Promotes urination and leaches

out dampness; clears heat from Heart Channel.
Common Formulas Used In: Dianthus.
Cautions in Use: Do not use this herb where there are deficient-cold symptoms.

81. Leonuris

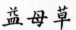

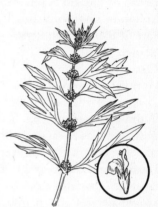

Latin Plant Name: Leonuri Hetero-phylli
Pinyin Mandarin Name: *Yi Mu Cao*
Common English Name: Chinese Motherwort
Part of Plant Used: Whole plant
Nature: Slightly cold
Taste: Acrid, bitter
Meridians Entered: Pericardium, Liver, Heart, Kidneys
Common Usages: This herb is used in formulas to treat acute-onset edema, especially with blood in urine; also used to treat high blood pressure, irregular menstruation with cramping and masses, and certain types of eczema; has also been used for retention of placenta. *(OM: Kidney imbalance; toxic Blood or Blood deficiency)*.
Traditional Usages and Functions: Invigorates Blood and regulates menstruation; invigorates Blood and reduces masses; promotes urination and reduces swelling.
Common Formulas Used In: Leonuris and Achyranthes.
Cautions in Use: Do not use during pregnancy. Do not use where there is deficient Yin or Blood.

82. Licorice

甘草

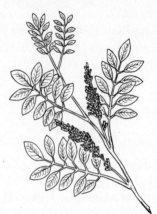

Latin Plant Name: Glycyrrhizae Uralensis
Pinyin Mandarin Name: *Gan Cao*
Common English Name: Licorice
Part of Plant Used: Root
Nature: Neutral
Taste: Sweet
Meridians Entered: All twelve Meridian Channels; particularly Lungs and Spleen
Common Usages: This herb is used in most formulas because of its excellent moderating and harmonizing influence on other herbs. It is also used as a tonic, and to treat spasms.

Traditional Usages and Functions: Tonifies Spleen and benefits Qi; moistens Lungs and stops coughing; clears heat and detoxifies fire poison; moderates and harmonizes the characteristics of other herbs; soothes spasms; soothes throat.

Common Formulas Used In: Agastache; Bupleurum, Inula, and Cyperus; Bupleurum and Tang Gui; Cimicafuga; Citrus and Pinellia; Clematis and Stephania; Cnidium and Tea; Corydalis; Fritillaria Extract Tablet; Gentiana; Ginseng and Astragalus; Ginseng and Atractylodes; Ginseng and Longan; Ginseng and Tang Gui; Hoelen and Polyporus; Lonicera and Forsythia; Ma Huang; Minor Bupleurum; Peony and Licorice; Pueraria Combination; Qiang-Huo and Turmeric; Stephania and Astragalus; Tang Gui and Ginseng Eight; Tu-Huo and Loranthus; Xanthium and Magnolia.

Cautions in Use: Do not use this herb where there is excessive dampness with nausea, bloating, or vomiting. Long-term use of this herb may cause high blood pressure and edema, and may lower rate of metabolism.

83. Ligusticum
川芎

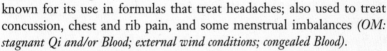

Latin Plant Name: Ligustici Wallichii
Pinyin Mandarin Name: *Chuan Xiong*
Common English Name: Ligusticum or
Cnidium
Part of Plant Used: Root
Nature: Warm
Taste: Acrid
Meridians Entered: Liver, Gallbladder,
Pericardium
Common Usages: This herb is well
known for its use in formulas that treat headaches; also used to treat
concussion, chest and rib pain, and some menstrual imbalances *(OM: stagnant Qi and/or Blood; external wind conditions; congealed Blood).*
Traditional Usages and Functions: Invigorates Blood and promotes
circulation of Qi ; expels Wind and alleviates pain. Used for headaches.
Common Formulas Used In: Angelica; Clematis and Stephania; Cnidium and Tea; Cyperus and Ligusticum; Ginseng and Tang Gui Ten;
Leonuris and Achyranthes; Tang Gui and Gardenia; Tang Gui and Ginseng Eight; Tang Gui Four; Tu-Huo and Loranthus.
Cautions in Use: Do not use during pregnancy. Do not use where
there is deficient Yin with heat, rising Liver Yang headaches, excessive
menstrual bleeding, or where there is very deficient Qi.

84. Ligustrum
女貞子

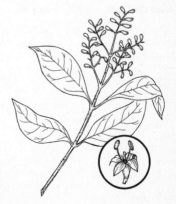

Latin Plant Name: Ligustri Lucidi
Pinyin Mandarin Name: *Nu Zhen Zi*
Common English Name: Ligustrum
Part of Plant Used: Fruit
Nature: Neutral
Taste: Sweet, bitter
Meridians Entered: Liver, Kidneys
Common Usages: This herb is used
in formulas to treat lower-back and
knee pain and/or weakness, leakage of

sperm, leukorrhea, weakened eyesight, gray hair, and ringing in the ears.

Traditional Usages and Functions: Nourishes and tonifies Liver and Kidneys.

Common Formulas Used In: Concha Marguerita and Ligustrum.

Cautions in Use: Do not use where there is deficient Yang, or with diarrhea from cold-deficient Spleen.

85. Linum

火麻仁

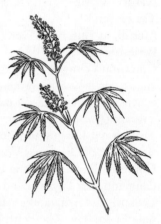

Latin Plant Name: Cannibis Sativae
Pinyin Mandarin Name: *Huo Ma Ren*
Common English Name: Cannibis Seed
Part of Plant Used: Seed
Nature: Neutral
Taste: Sweet
Meridians Entered: Spleen, Stomach, Large Intestine
Common Usages: This herb is used in formulas to treat constipation *(OM: caused by chronic Yin Deficiency)*, and is sometimes used topically (or in herbal combinations) to promote healing of sores.

Traditional Usages and Functions: Nourishes and moistens Intestines; nourishes Yin; clears heat and promotes healing of sores.

Common Formulas Used In: Apricot Seed and Linum.

Cautions in Use: Do not use where there is diarrhea.

86. Longan (Arillis)

龍眼肉

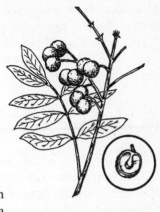

Latin Plant Name: Arillis Euphoriae
Longanae
Pinyin Mandarin Name: *Long Yan Rou*
Common English Name: Longan Fruit
Part of Plant Used: Fruit
Nature: Warm
Taste: Sweet
Meridians Entered: Heart, Spleen
Common Usages: This herb is used in
formulas to treat certain types of insomnia
(OM: due to deficient Heart or Spleen weakness), frequently caused by post-
birth weakness where mother has not had sufficient time to recover.
Traditional Usages and Functions: Tonifies Heart and Spleen, nour-
ishes Blood, and calms Spirit.
Common Formulas Used In: Ginseng and Longan.
Cautions in Use: Do not use where there is fire and stagnation of
phlegm and dampness.

87. Lonicera Flower

金銀花

Latin Plant Name: Lonicerae Japonicae
Pinyin Mandarin Name: *Jin Yin Hua*
Common English Name: Honeysuckle
Flower
Part of Plant Used: Flower
Nature: Cold
Taste: Sweet
Meridians Entered: Lungs, Stomach,
Large Intestine
Common Usages: This herb is used in
formulas to treat heat-related symptoms of sores, hot diarrhea, burning
urine, and external respiratory symptoms with swollen tonsils and yel-
low, scanty phlegm.
Traditional Usages and Functions: Clears heat and detoxifies fire
poison; clears damp heat; expels externally contracted wind heat.

Common Formulas Used In: Ilex and Evodia; Lonicera and For-sythia; Rhubarb and Scutellaria.
Cautions in Use: Do not use where there is diarrhea from cold, Defi-ciency of Spleen and Stomach, or with deficiency sores or ulcers with-out redness or heat.

88. Loranthus

桑寄生

Latin Plant Name: Loranthi seu Visci
Pinyin Mandarin Name: *Sang Ji Sheng*
Common English Name: Loranthus
Part of Plant Used: Stems
Nature: Neutral
Taste: Bitter, sweet
Meridians Entered: Liver, Kidneys
Common Usages: This herb is used in
formulas to treat lower-back pain and weakness often accompanied by
atrophy; to strengthen tendons; to prevent miscarriage *(OM: by nour-ishing Blood and calming the fetus);* and to treat high blood pressure.
Traditional Usages and Functions: Tonifies Liver and Kidneys and
expels wind dampness; nourishes Blood and calms the Womb; nour-ishes Blood and makes the skin glow.
Common Formulas Used In: Tian Qi and Eucommia; Tu-Huo and
Loranthus.
Cautions in Use: None.

89. Lotus Seed

蓮子

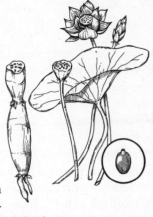

Latin Plant Name: Nelumbinis
Pinyin Mandarin Name: *Lian Zi*
Common English Name: Lotus Seed
Part of Plant Used: Seed
Nature: Neutral
Taste: Sweet, astringent
Meridians Entered: Heart, Spleen, Kidneys
Common Usages: This herb is used in formulas to treat insomnia and palpitations *(OM: deficiency often accompanied by heat signs).*
Traditional Usages and Functions: Clears fire and nourishes Kidneys; strengthens Spleen and stops diarrhea.
Common Formulas Used In: Ginseng and Atractylodes.
Cautions in Use: Do not use where there is abdominal bloating or constipation.

90. Lumbricus

地龍

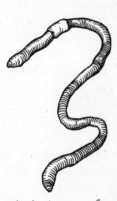

Latin Plant Name: Lumbricus
Pinyin Mandarin Name: *Di Long*
Common English Name: Earthworm
Part Used: Whole
Nature: Cold
Taste: Salty
Meridians Entered: Liver, Spleen, Lung
Common Usages: Lumbricus is used in formulas to treat spasms, asthma, and high fever, to assist in recovery from strokes, and to drain water; also used to treat high blood pressure, arthritis pain and stiffness, and tics *(OM: wind symptoms).*
Traditional Usages and Functions: Quells heat and stops spasms; expels wind and activates channels; promotes urination; stops wheezing.
Common Formulas Used In: Prunella and Scutellaria.
Cautions in Use: Do not use during pregnancy. Use with caution where there are no true heat symptoms.

91. Lycium
枸杞子

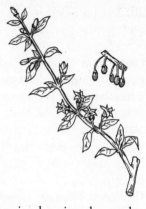

Latin Plant Name: Lycii Chinensis
Pinyin Mandarin Name: *Gou Qi Zi*
Common English Name: Lycium Fruit
Part of Plant Used: Fruit
Nature: Neutral
Taste: Sweet
Meridians Entered: Liver, Kidneys
Common Usages: This herb is used in formulas to treat visual disturbances such as sensitivity to light, blurred vision, and poor visual acuity; also used to treat general weakness, diabetic symptoms, chronic Lung disorders, impotence.
Traditional Usages and Functions: Nourishes and tonifies Liver and Kidneys; benefits Essence and brightens eyes.
Common Formulas Used In: Cerebral Tonic Pills; Rehmannia and Dogwood Fruit.
Cautions in Use: Do not use where there is deficient Spleen and dampness, or if there is an external excess heat imbalance. Use cautiously where there is an internal heat imbalance.

92. Lysimachia (Desmodium)
金錢草

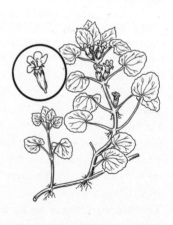

Latin Plant Name: Glechoma Longituba
Pinyin Mandarin Name: *Jin Qian Cao*
Common English Name: Lysimachia, Desmodium, or other names relative to locale
Part of Plant Used: Whole plant
Nature: Neutral
Taste: Sweet, bland, slightly salty
Meridians Entered: Lungs, Liver, Gallbladder
Common Usages: This herb is used in formulas to treat stones in urinary or bile tracts, and to treat symptoms of stones including

inflammation, spasm, and swelling of surrounding tissue; also reputed to be useful in treating snakebites, jaundice, abscesses, and traumatic injury.

Traditional Usages and Functions: Expels stones; clears heat and promotes urination; clears Liver Channel heat; detoxifies poison and reduces swelling.

Common Formulas Used In: Rhubarb and Scutellaria.

Cautions in Use: Do not use for excessive periods of time due to the herb's diuretic effect.

93. Magnetitum

磁石

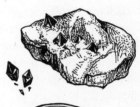

Latin Plant Name: Magnetitum
Pinyin Mandarin Name: *Ci Shi*
Common English Name: Magnetic Stone
Part of Plant Used: Whole plant
Nature: Cold
Taste: Acrid
Meridians Entered: Kidneys, Liver
Common Usages: This herb is used in formulas to treat various symptoms of irritability including tremors, palpitations, restlessness, insomnia, or convulsions; also used to treat dizziness, vertigo, blurry vision and ringing in the ears *(OM: associated with Liver and/or Kidney imbalance)*; also has been found useful in treating certain types of asthma.

Traditional Usages and Functions: Settles and tranquilizes Spirit; pacifies Liver and restrains floating Yang; aids Kidneys in grasping Qi.

Common Formulas Used In: Rehmannia and Magnetitum.

Cautions in Use: None.

94. Magnolia Bark

厚樸

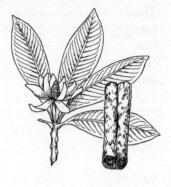

Latin Plant Name: Magnoliae Officinalis
Pinyin Mandarin Name: *Hou Po*
Common English Name: Magnolia Bark
Part of Plant Used: Bark
Nature: Warm
Taste: Bitter, acrid, aromatic
Meridians Entered: Spleen, Stomach, Lungs, Large Intestine
Common Usages: This herb is used in formulas to treat abdominal bloating, flatulence, nausea, diarrhea, and indigestion *(OM: dampness and stagnation);* also used in formulas to treat asthma and coughing, and to break up congestion caused by excessive phlegm that accompanies wheezing.
Traditional Usages and Functions: Moves Qi, transforms dampness and resolves stagnation; warms and transforms phlegm and directs Rebellious Qi downward.
Common Formulas Used In: Agastache; Apricot Seed and Linum; Bupleurum, Inula, and Cyperus.
Cautions in Use: Use cautiously during pregnancy. Do not use with Yin- or Qi-deficiency imbalances.

95. Magnolia Flower

辛荑花

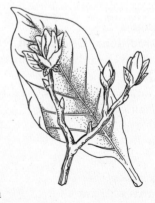

Latin Plant Name: Magnolia Liliflorae
Pinyin Mandarin Name: *Xin Yi Hua*
Common English Name: Magnolia Flower
Part of Plant Used: Flower
Nature: Slightly warm
Taste: Acrid
Meridians Entered: Lungs
Common Usages: This herb is used in formulas to treat symptoms of sinus infection and inflammation, congestion, and headache.

Traditional Usages and Functions: Expels wind and opens nasal passages.
Common Formulas Used In: Xanthium and Magnolia.
Cautions in Use: Use cautiously where there is dehydration with Yin deficiency.

96. Marguerite Concha
珍珠母

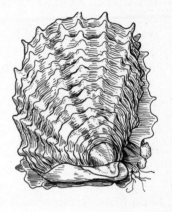

Latin Plant Name: Margaritaferae, Concha
Pinyin Mandarin Name: *Zhen Zhu Mu*
Common English Name: Mother-of-Pearl
Part of Plant Used: Whole shell
Nature: Cold
Taste: Sweet, salty
Meridians Entered: Liver, Heart
Common Usages: This herb is used in formulas to treat dizziness, vertigo, ringing in the ears, acid stomach, cataracts, insomnia, seizures, or night blindness.
Traditional Usages and Functions: Pacifies Liver, brightens eyes, and calms Spirit.
Common Formulas Used In: Concha Marguerita and Ligustrum.
Cautions in Use: Use cautiously where there is a sensation of coldness in the abdomen.

97. Massa Fermenta
(preparation)
神曲

Latin Plant Name: Massa Fermentata
Pinyin Mandarin Name: *Shenqu*
Common English Name: Divine Fermented Mass
Part of Plant Used: A preparation of Artemesia, Apricot Seed, Xanthium, wheat flour, polygonum, or phaseolus combined and fermented together.

Nature: Warm
Taste: Sweet, acrid
Meridians Entered: Spleen, Stomach
Common Usages: This herbal preparation is used in formulas to treat digestive problems including symptoms of diarrhea with a sensation of fullness and swelling in upper abdomen, poor appetite, indigestion from poor digestion of starches, bloating, headache, and mild food poisoning.
Traditional Usages and Functions: Dissolves stagnation of food and harmonizes Stomach.
Common Formulas Used In: Cyperus and Ligusticum.
Cautions in Use: Use cautiously during pregnancy. Do not use where there is Stomach fire.

98. Moutan
牡丹皮

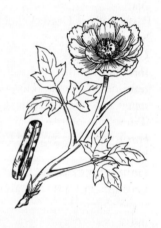

Latin Plant Name: Moutan Radicis
Pinyin Mandarin Name: *Mu Dan Pi*
Common English Name: Moutan
Part of Plant Used: Small curls of root bark
Nature: Cool
Taste: Acrid, bitter
Meridians Entered: Heart, Liver, Kidneys
Common Usages: This herb is used in formulas to treat gynecological problems including tumors, masses, lumps in abdomen, or irregular or missing menses, after actual malignancy has been ruled out *(OM: Blood stasis)*; also used for skin eruptions, mouth sores, abnormal bleeding from the nose, and blood in sputum, vomit, or under the skin with or following a high fever; also has been used to treat intestinal abscesses, such as appendicitis, by reducing swelling and draining pus.
Traditional Usages and Functions: Clears heat and cools Blood; clears deficiency fire, invigorates Blood and dispels congealed Blood; clears ascending Liver fire; drains pus and reduces swelling.
Common Formulas Used In: Anemarrhena, Phellodendron, and Rehmannia; Bupleurum, Inula, and Cyperus; Eight Immortal Long

Life Pill; Leonuris and Achyranthes; Rehmannia and Dogwood Fruit; Rehmannia and Magnetitum; Rehmannia Eight; Rehmannia Six.
Cautions in Use: Do not use during pregnancy. Do not use where there are cold conditions, excessive menstrual bleeding, or deficient Yin with excessive sweating.

99. Myrrh Gum
没藥

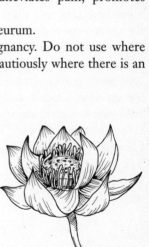

Latin Plant Name: Myrrha
Pinyin Mandarin Name: *Mo Yao*
Common English Name: Myrrh Gum
Part of Plant Used: Gum resin
Nature: Neutral
Taste: Bitter
Meridians Entered: Heart, Liver
Common Usages: This herb is used in formulas to treat pain associated with trauma or internal imbalances *(OM: Blood stasis);* also used topically to speed regeneration of tissue.
Traditional Usages and Functions: Invigorates Blood and dispels congealed Blood, reduces swelling and alleviates pain; promotes healing.
Common Formulas Used In: Minor Bupleurum.
Cautions in Use: Do not use during pregnancy. Do not use where there is excessive menstrual bleeding. Use cautiously where there is an internal heat imbalance.

100. Nelumbinus Stamen
蓮鬚

Latin Plant Name: Nelumbinus
Pinyin Mandarin Name: *Lian Xu*
Common English Name: Lotus Stamen
Part of Plant Used: Stamen
Nature: Neutral
Taste: Sweet, astringent
Meridians Entered: Kidneys, Heart

Common Usages: This herb is used in formulas that treat severe incontinence, frequent urination, and chronic leukorrhea; also used to stop bleeding and to treat seminal emissions (in combination with lotus seed).

Traditional Usages and Functions: Stabilizes Kidneys; retains Essence.

Common Formulas Used In: Hoelen and Polyporus.

Remarks: Lotus stamen provides stronger astringency action than does lotus seed.

Cautions in Use: Do not use where there is difficult urination.

101. Notoptergi
羌活

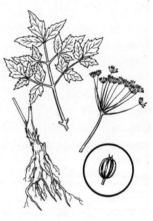

Latin Plant Name: Notopterygii
Pinyin Mandarin Name: *Qiang-Huo* or *Chiang-Huo*
Common English Name: Notoptergi
Part of Plant Used: Root
Nature: Warm
Taste: Acrid, bitter, aromatic
Meridians Entered: Bladder, Kidneys
Common Usages: This herb is used in formulas to treat pain associated with flu-like symptoms including headaches, joint pain—especially in upper back and limbs, and the pain of sinus congestion *(OM: surface/exterior conditions)*; also used to treat painful sores and inflammations.

Traditional Usages and Functions: Releases exterior and disperses cold; penetrates through painful obstruction and alleviates pain; guides Qi to Greater Yang and Governing Channels.

Common Formulas Used In: Clematis and Stephania; Cnidium and Tea; Qiang-Huo and Turmeric.

Cautions in Use: Do not use where there is deficient Blood or Yin, or where there is a deficient exterior imbalance.

102. Ophiopogon

麥門冬

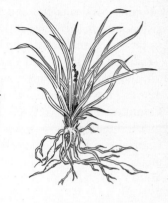

Latin Plant Name: Ophiopogonis
Japonici
Pinyin Mandarin Name: *Mai Men Dong*
Common English Name: Ophiopogon
Part of Plant Used: Root
Nature: Slightly cold
Taste: Sweet, slightly bitter
Meridians Entered: Lungs, Stomach,
Heart
Common Usages: This herb is used in formulas to treat constipation, thick sputum—sometimes tinged with blood, scanty urine, thirst, dry throat, mouth sores, symptoms of diabetic imbalance, restlessness, and chronic bronchitis *(OM: interior dryness and Yin deficiency, especially in Lungs, Heart, and Intestines)*.
Traditional Usages and Functions: Nourishes Yin and clears heat; moistens Lungs and stops coughing; moistens Intestines.
Common Formulas Used In: Eight Immortal Long Life Pill; Ginseng and Zizyphus.
Cautions in Use: Do not use where there is cold-deficient diarrhea with a sensation of coldness in the abdomen, or where there are symptoms of congested fluids such as bloating and indigestion with a feeling of fullness.

103. Oyster Shell

牡蠣

Latin Plant Name: Concha Ostreae
Pinyin Mandarin Name: *Mu Li*
Common English Name: Oyster Shell
Part of Plant Used: Whole shell
(crushed)
Nature: Cool
Taste: Salty, astringent
Meridians Entered: Liver, Kidneys
Common Usages: Oyster shell is used in
formulas to treat irritability with associated symptoms of palpitations,

insomnia, and anxiety, and sometimes ringing in the ears, blurred vision, and flushed face *(OM: Yin deficiency)*; also used to treat night sweats, nocturnal emissions, heartburn, and goiter.

Traditional Usages and Functions: Settles and calms Spirit; benefits Yin and restrains floating Yang; prevents leakage of fluids; softens hardness and dissipates nodules; absorbs acidity and alleviates pain.

Common Formulas Used In: Bupleurum and Dragon Bone; Tang Gui and Indigo.

Cautions in Use: Do not use where there is high fever with no sweating.

104. Peony Alba

白芍

Latin Plant Name: Paeoniae Lactiflorae
Pinyin Mandarin Name: *Bai Shao*
Common English Name: White Peony
Part of Plant Used: Root
Nature: Cool
Taste: Bitter, sour
Meridians Entered: Liver, Spleen
Common Usages: This herb has strong Blood-toning actions and is used in formulas that treat various blood imbalances including most menstrual disorders, poor circulation, and heat rashes; also used to stop bleeding and prevent miscarriages *(OM: deficient Blood and Liver function)*.

Traditional Usages and Functions: Nourishes Blood, activates circulation, and cools Blood; has astringent actions; pacifies Liver and alleviates pain; restrains Yin and adjusts Nutritive and Protective levels.

Common Formulas Used In: Apricot Seed and Linum; Bupleurum, Inula, and Cyperus; Bupleurum and Tang Gui; Clematis and Stephania; Corydalis; Ginseng and Tang Gui Ten; Peony and Licorice; Pueraria Combination; Rehmannia and Dogwood Fruit; Tang Gui and Gardenia; Tang Gui and Ginseng Eight; Tang Gui Four; Tu-Huo and Loranthus.

Cautions in Use: Do not use where there is cold-deficiency diarrhea.

105. Peony Rubra
赤芍

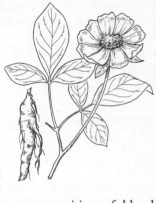

Latin Plant Name: Paeoniae Rubra
Pinyin Mandarin Name: *Chi Shao*
Common English Name: Red Peony
Part of Plant Used: Root
Nature: Slightly cold
Taste: Sour, bitter
Meridians Entered: Liver, Spleen
Common Usages: This herb is used in formulas to treat symptoms of skin erup-
tions, trauma, red swollen eyes, bloody nose, vomiting of blood, absence of menses, rashes, and acne *(OM: Blood stasis and heat conditions)*; also used to reduce pain *(OM: stagnant Blood and Liver Fire)*.
Traditional Usages and Functions: Invigorates Blood and dispels congealed Blood; clears Heat and cools Blood; clears Liver Fire.
Common Formulas Used In: Qiang-Huo and Turmeric.
Cautions in Use: Use cautiously where there is a Blood deficiency.

106. Peppermint
薄荷

Latin Plant Name: Mentha Arvensis
Pinyin Mandarin Name: *Bo He*
Common English Name: Peppermint
Part of plant used: Whole plant
Nature: Cooling
Taste: Acrid, aromatic
Meridians Entered: Liver, Lungs
Common Usages: This herb is used in formulas to treat sore throats, skin ail-
ments on the upper body, itching, rashes, measles, pinkeye (conjunctivitis), and headache; may also be used to treat some menstrual imbalances, with the sensation of pressure in the sides of the ribs, and emotional instability *(OM: stagnant Liver Qi)*.
Traditional Usages and Functions: Disperses wind heat; clears head and eyes and benefits throat; encourages rashes to surface; allows constrained Liver Qi to flow freely.

Common Formulas Used In: Bupleurum and Tang Gui; Cnidium and Tea; Ilex and Evodia; Lonicera and Forsythia.

Remarks: When preparing as a tea, add to liquid during the last few minutes of boiling.

Cautions in Use: Do not use where there is a deficient exterior imbalance, or where there is deficient Yin with heat.

107. Perilla Leaf

紫蘇葉

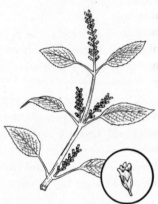

Latin Plant Name: Perillae
Frutescentis

Pinyin Mandarin Name: *Zi Su Ye*

Common English Name: Perilla
Leaf

Part of Plant Used: Leaf

Nature: Warm

Taste: Acrid, aromatic

Meridians Entered: Lungs, Spleen

Common Usages: This herb is used in formulas to treat asthma, especially where there is a weak constitution leading to digestive disturbances that include belching, sneezing, weak coughing, and phlegm; also used to prevent miscarriage and to treat morning sickness, especially with belching.

Traditional Usages and Functions: Releases exterior and disperses cold; circulates Qi and harmonizes Middle Burner; calms fetus; alleviates seafood poisoning.

Common Formulas Used In: Agastache.

Cautions in Use: Do not use where there is an exterior deficiency condition with excess sweating, or where there are damp-heat imbalances.

108. Phellodendron

黄柏

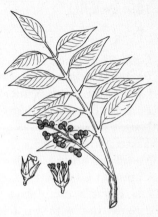

Latin Plant Name: Phellodendri
Pinyin Mandarin Name: *Huang Bai*
Common English Name: Phelloden-
dron
Part of Plant Used: Bark
Nature: Cold
Taste: Bitter
Meridians Entered: Kidneys, Bladder
Common Usages: This herb is used in
formulas to treat burning and fetid diar-
rhea with jaundice, fever, urinary-tract

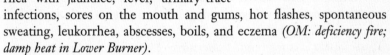

infections, sores on the mouth and gums, hot flashes, spontaneous
sweating, leukorrhea, abscesses, boils, and eczema *(OM: deficiency fire;
damp heat in Lower Burner)*.

Phellodendron's antiseptic qualities make it useful as an anti-inflam-
matory treatment for most inflammatory conditions in body, from
pelvic inflammatory disease to skin and mouth lesions.

Traditional Usages and Functions: Drains damp heat, particularly
in the Lower Burner; quells Kidney fire; drains fire and detoxifies fire
poison.

Common Formulas Used In: Anemarrhena, Phellodendron, and
Rehmannia; Hoelen and Polyporus; Tang Gui and Gardenia; Xanthium
and Magnolia.

Cautions in Use: Do not use where there is deficient Spleen, diarrhea,
or a weak stomach.

109. Pinellia
半夏

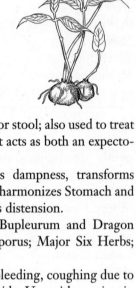

Latin Plant Name: Pinelliae Ternatae
Pinyin Mandarin Name: *Ban Xia*
Common English Name: Pinellia
Part of Plant Used: Root
Nature: Warm
Taste: Acrid, poisonous
Meridians Entered: Spleen, Stomach
Common Usages: This herb is used in formulas to treat excess fluids or phlegm in the digestive tract with symptoms such as nausea, vomiting, and diarrhea, with phlegm in vomit or stool; also used to treat excess clear or white phlegm in lungs, where it acts as both an expectorant and a dispersant.
Traditional Usages and Functions: Dries dampness, transforms phlegm, and causes Rebellious Qi to descend; harmonizes Stomach and stops vomiting; dissipates nodules and reduces distension.
Common Formulas Used In: Agastache; Bupleurum and Dragon Bone; Citrus and Pinellia; Hoelen and Polyporus; Major Six Herbs; Minor Bupleurum.
Cautions in Use: Do not use where there is bleeding, coughing due to deficient Yin, or where there are depleted fluids. Use with caution in heat imbalances.

110. Plantago Seed
車前子

Latin Plant Name: Plantaginis
Pinyin Mandarin Name: *Che Qian Zi*
Common English Name: Plantago Seed
Part of Plant Used: Seed
Nature: Cold
Taste: Sweet, bland
Meridians Entered: Kidney, Bladder, Liver, Lung, Small Intestine
Common Usages: This herb is used in formulas to treat urinary-tract

burning, redness, and itching; eye pain, burning, itching, or dryness; high blood pressure; excessive colored phlegm; and diarrhea *(OM: damp-heat conditions)*. Also used as a diuretic.

Traditional Usages and Functions: Promotes urination and clears heat; clears the eyes; expels Phlegm and stops coughing.

Common Formulas Used In: Dianthus; Gentiana.

Remarks: When boiling plantago seeds for tea, wrap them in cheese-cloth.

Cautions in Use: Use carefully where there is exhausted Yang Qi, or where there is sperm leakage due to Kidney deficiency or overwork.

111. Platycodon

桔梗

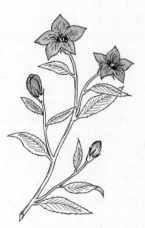

Latin Plant Name: Platycodi Grandiflori
Pinyin Mandarin Name: *Jie Geng*
Common English Name: Platycodon
Part of Plant Used: Root
Nature: Neutral
Taste: Bitter, acrid
Meridians Entered: Lungs, Stomach
Common Usages: This neutral herb is used in many cold and flu formulas to enhance expectoration and expel pus from abscesses in Lungs or throat; also used to treat laryngitis *(OM: Lung or skin imbalances; hot or cold conditions)*.

Traditional Usages and Functions: Circulates Lung Qi and expels Phlegm; promotes Yin; promotes discharge of pus; benefits throat; directs the effect of other herbs upward; tonifies and sedates.

Common Formulas Used In: Agastache; Fritillaria Extract Tablet; Ginseng and Atractylodes; Ginseng and Zizyphus; Lonicera and Forsythia; Xanthium and Magnolia.

Cautions in Use: Do not use where there is Blood in the sputum (as in tuberculosis). Do not use in large quantities, as it may cause nausea and vomiting.

112. Polygala
遠志

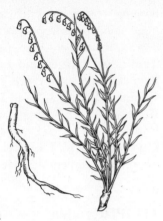

Latin Plant Name: Polygalae Tenuifoliae
Pinyin Mandarin Name: *Yuan Zi*
Common English Name: Polygala
Part of Plant Used: Root
Nature: Warm
Taste: Bitter, acrid
Meridians Entered: Kidneys, Heart, Lungs
Common Usages: This herb is used in formulas to treat restlessness, anxiety, and insomnia; also used to clear phlegm from Lungs and to treat acute and chronic bronchitis.
Traditional Usages and Functions: Calms Spirit, centers mind, and facilitates flow of Qi in the Heart; tonifies Heart Qi, Blood, and Yin; expels Phlegm and clears orifices; expels Phlegm from Lungs.
Common Formulas Used In: Cerebral Tonic Pills; Fritillaria Extract Tablet; Ginseng and Longan; Ginseng and Zizyphus.
Cautions in Use: Do not use where there is deficient Yin with heat signs.

113. Polygonum Multiflorum
何首烏

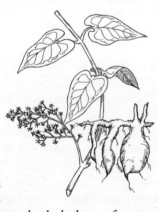

Latin Plant Name: Polygoni Multiflori
Pinyin Mandarin Name: *He Shou Wu*
Common English Name: Polygonatum
Part of Plant Used: Root
Nature: Slightly warm
Taste: Bitter, sweet, astringent
Meridians Entered: Liver, Kidney
Common Usages: This herb is used in formulas to treat symptoms of chronic disease, including general weakness, weak lower back, leakage of sperm, leukorrhea, dizziness, blurred vision, insomnia, anemia, constipation, poor appetite, fatigue, and weight loss; also used to treat skin lumps, sores, abscesses, and boils; may also be used to restore hair color and restore skin tone and color.

Traditional Usages and Functions: Tonifies Liver and Kidneys, nourishes Blood, and benefits Essence; retains Essence and stops leakage; detoxifies fire poison; moistens Intestines and moves stool; expels wind from skin by nourishing Blood.
Common Formulas Used In: Polygonum Tablet.
Cautions in Use: Do not use where there is deficient Spleen or excessive phlegm.

114. Poria
茯苓

Latin Plant Name: Poria Cocos
Pinyin Mandarin Name: *Fu Ling*
Common English Name: Poria
Part of Plant Used: Fungus adhering to
a specific pine tree
Nature: Neutral
Taste: Sweet, bland
Meridians Entered: Heart, Spleen, Lungs
Common Usages: This herb is used in formulas to treat fluid and phlegm congestion where there is poor metabolism—particularly in digestive system—with symptoms of poor appetite, fatigue, diarrhea, bloating, scanty urine, palpitations, insomnia, headache, dizziness, and forgetfulness; also use to treat coughs and asthma, anxiety, and related insomnia.
Traditional Usages and Functions: Promotes urination and leaches out dampness; strengthens Spleen and harmonizes Middle Burner; strengthens Spleen and transforms Phlegm; quiets Heart and calms Spirit.
Common Formulas Used In: Agastache; Anemarrhena, Phellodendron, and Rehmannia; Bupleurum and Dragon Bone; Bupleurum and Tang Gui; Citrus and Pinellia; Clematis and Stephania; Eight Immortal Long Life Pill; Ginseng and Atractylodes; Ginseng and Longan; Ginseng and Tang Gui Ten; Hoelen and Polyporus; Hoelen Five; Major Four Herbs; Major Six Herbs; Rehmannia and Dogwood Fruit; Rehmannia and Magnetitum; Rehmannia Eight; Rehmannia Six; Tang Gui and Ginseng Eight; Tu-Huo and Loranthus.
Cautions in Use: Do not use where there are deficient-cold symptoms or excessive urination.

115. Prunella

夏枯草

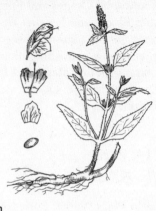

Latin Plant Name: Prunellae Vulgaris
Pinyin Mandarin Name: *Xia Ku Cao*
Common English Name: Selfheal
Part of Plant Used: Whole or broken flowering spike
Nature: Cold
Taste: Sweet, acrid, slightly bitter
Meridians Entered: Liver, Gallbladder, Lungs
Common Usages: This herb is used in formulas to treat swollen lymph glands, goiter, tumors, abscesses, high blood pressure, and vertigo *(OM: swellings due to Liver fire and constraint);* also used to treat headaches; and eye pain, swelling, and redness *(OM: Liver fire).*
Traditional Usages and Functions: Clears Liver and brightens eyes; clears heat and dissipates nodules.
Common Formulas Used In: Leonuris and Achyranthes; Prunella and Scutellaria.
Cautions in Use: Do not use where there is deficient Spleen or Stomach imbalances.

116. Pseudoginseng

田七

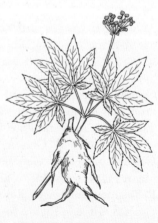

Latin Plant Name: Pseudoginseng
Pinyin Mandarin Name: *San Qi* or *Tian Qi*
Common English Name: Pseudoginseng Root
Part of Plant Used: Root
Nature: Slightly warm
Taste: Sweet, slightly bitter
Meridians Entered: Liver, Stomach, Large Intestine
Common Usages: This herb is used singly or in formulas to treat most types of bleeding, including bleeding from bruising, injury, blood clots,

miscarriage, childbirth, and excessive menstrual flow; also used to break up blood clots *(OM: congealed Blood)*.

Traditional Usages and Functions: Stops bleeding and transforms congealed Blood; reduces swelling and alleviates pain.

Common Formulas Used In: Pseudoginseng and Dragon Blood; Tian Qi and Eucommia.

Cautions in Use: Do not use during pregnancy. Use with caution where there is deficient Blood.

117. Pueraria

葛根

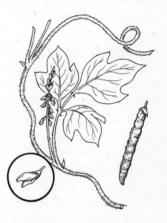

Latin Plant Name: Puerariae
Pinyin Mandarin Name: *Ge Gen*
Common English Name: Kudzu Root
Part of Plant Used: Root
Nature: Cool
Taste: Sweet, acrid
Meridians Entered: Spleen, Stomach

Common Usages: This herb is used in formulas to treat shoulder and neck tightness, fever, sore throat, thirst, sinus congestion, and headache *(OM: exterior ailments)*; also used to treat diabetic syndrome, nausea, vomiting, diarrhea *(OM: deficient Fluids)*, and high blood pressure with upper-back tightness and headache.

Traditional Usages and Functions: Releases muscles and clears Heat; nourishes Fluids and alleviates thirst; encourages the rash of measles to surface; alleviates diarrhea.

Common Formulas Used In: Pueraria Combination.

Cautions in Use: Use caution where there is excessive sweating or a sensation of coldness in the Stomach.

118. Rehmannia (raw)

生地黄

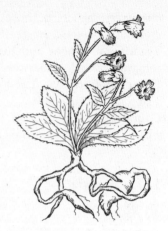

Latin Plant Name: Rehmanniae Gluti-nosae
Pinyin Mandarin Name: *Sheng Di Huang*
Common English Name: Chinese Fox-glove Root
Part of Plant Used: Root
Nature: Cold
Taste: Sweet, bitter
Meridians Entered: Liver, Kidneys, Heart

Common Usages: This herb is used in formulas to treat symptoms of high fever, thirst, mouth and tongue sores, irritability, flushing of the cheeks, dry stool, lower-back pain, nosebleed, insomnia, blood in the urine, uterine bleeding, afternoon or low-grade fevers, hemorrhage, and diabetic syndrome *(OM: Blood heat symptoms).*

Traditional Usages and Functions: Clears heat and cools Blood; nourishes Yin and Blood and generates Fluids; cools upward blazing of Heart Fire. By raising Yin and increasing production of Fluids, this herb also settles Yang, thus reducing heat in a more stable way than by simply extinguishing Fire. Used for Wasting and Thirsting Syndrome.

Common Formulas Used In: Concha Marguerita and Ligustrum; Gentiana; Ginseng and Zizyphus; Clematis and Stephania; Leonuris and Achyranthes.

Cautions in Use: Do not use during pregnancy. Do not use where there are damp phlegm imbalances, deficient Spleen imbalances with dampness or deficient Yang, or deficient Blood or Stomach imbalances.

119. Rehmannia (steamed)

熟地黄

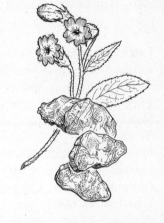

Latin Plant Name: Rehmanniae Glutinosae Conquitae
Pinyin Mandarin Name: *Shu Di Huang*
Common English Name: Steamed Chinese Foxglove
Part of Plant Used: Root cooked in wine
Nature: Warm
Taste: Sweet
Meridians Entered: Liver, Kidneys, Heart

Common Usages: This Blood- and Yin-tonifying herb is used in formulas to treat symptoms of pallid face, palpitations, insomnia, irregular menstruation, excessive menstrual and postchildbirth bleeding; also used to treat night sweating, nocturnal emissions, and diabetic syndrome; dizziness and palpitation (*OM: due to Blood deficiency*), and lower-back pain.

Traditional Usages and Functions: Tonifies Blood; nourishes Yin.

Common Formulas Used In: Anemarrhena, Phellodendron, and Rehmannia; Eight Immortal Long Life Pill; Ginseng and Tang Gui Ten; Rehmannia and Dogwood Fruit; Rehmannia and Magnetitum; Rehmannia Eight; Rehmannia Six; Tang Gui and Gardenia; Tan Gui and Ginseng Eight; Tang Gui Four; Tu-Huo and Loranthus.

Cautions in Use: Use with caution where there is deficient Spleen and Stomach, or where there is stagnant Qi or phlegm leading to diarrhea or indigestion.

120. Rhubarb

大黄

Latin Plant Name: Rheum Palmatum
Pinyin Mandarin Name: *Da Huang*
Common English Name: Rhubarb
Part of Plant Used: Root
Nature: Cold
Taste: Bitter
Meridians Entered: Stomach, Large
Intestine, Liver

Common Usages: This herb is used in formulas to treat symptoms of high fever, excessive sweating, thirst, constipation, bloating, pain, jaundice, high blood pressure, hemmorhage, no menstruation, immobile abdominal masses, and hot, swollen, painful eyes *(OM: internal-heat/damp-heat conditions and stagnant Blood);* also used to treat skin burns, worms, edema and delirium.

Traditional Usages and Functions: Drains heat and moves stool; drains damp heat; drains excess heat from Blood; invigorates Blood and breaks up congealed Blood; clears heat obstructing Blood level; clears heat and detoxifies fire poison.

Common Formulas Used In: Apricot Seed and Linum; Bupleurum and Dragon Bone; Cimicafuga; Dianthus; Leonuris and Achyranthes; Rhubarb and Scutellaria.

Cautions in Use: Use with caution during pregnancy and immediately after birth. Do not use where there are exterior imbalances, deficient Qi or Blood, or cold-deficient Spleen and Stomach.

121. Salvia

丹参

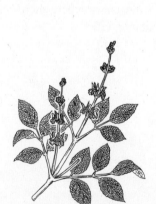

Latin Plant Name: Salviae Miltiorrhizae
Pinyin Mandarin Name: *Dan Shen*
Common English Name: Salvia
Part of Plant Used: Root
Nature: Slightly cold
Taste: Bitter
Meridians Entered: Heart, Pericardium,
Liver

Common Usages: This herb is used in formulas to treat symptoms of tumors, acne, boils, skin sores, menstrual irregularity and absence, endometriosis, fibroids, insomnia, irritability, or palpitations *(OM: Blood stasis with heat);* also used for its tranquilizing effects, and to treat coronary heart disease in combination with other specific herbs.

Traditional Usages and Functions: Invigorates Blood and breaks up congealed Blood; clears heat and soothes irritability.

Common Formulas Used In: Concha Marguerita and Ligustrum; Ginseng and Zizyphus.

Cautions in Use: Do not use during pregnancy. Use with caution where there are no symptoms of congealed Blood.

122. Sandalwood

檀香

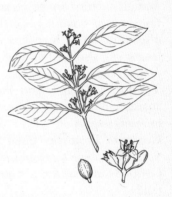

Latin Plant Name: Santali Albi
Pinyin Mandarin Name: *Tan Xiang*
Common English Name: Sandal-wood
Part of Plant Used: Heart of the wood
Nature: Warm
Taste: Acrid, bitter
Meridians Entered: Spleen, Stomach, Lungs, Heart
Common Usages: This herb is used in formulas that treat pain, especially pain in the Stomach *(OM: due to stagnation and cold)* and pain in the chest (angina) *(OM: due to Blood stasis)*, when also under the care of a practitioner.

Traditional Usages and Functions: Moves Qi and alleviates pain.

Common Formulas Used In: Bupleurum, Inula, and Cyperus.

Cautions in Use: Do not use where there is a Yin deficiency with heat.

123. Saussurea
木香

Latin Plant Name: Saussureae seu
Vladimiriae
Pinyin Mandarin Name: *Mu Xiang*
Common English Name: Saussurea
Part of Plant Used: Root
Nature: Warm
Taste: Acrid, bitter
Meridians Entered: Spleen, Stomach,
Large Intestine, Gallbladder, Liver
Common Usages: This herb is used in
formulas to treat symptoms such as abdominal and chest pains, indigestion, nausea, vomiting, diarrhea (or urge to defecate with no results, often with spasm), bronchial asthma, weak digestion, and bloating *(OM: stagnation);* also used to treat jaundice, and infections in the bronchial, vaginal, and intestinal areas.
Traditional Usages and Functions: Moves Qi and alleviates pain; adjusts and regulates Stagnant Qi in Intestines; strengthens Spleen and prevents stagnation.
Common Formulas Used In: Ginseng and Longan; Rhubarb and Scutellaria; Tang Gui and Indigo.
Cautions in Use: Do not use where there is deficient Yin or depleted fluids.

124. Schisandra
五味子

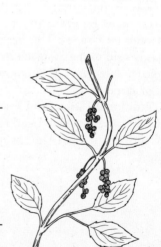

Latin Plant Name: Schizandrae Chinensis
Pinyin Mandarin Name: *Wu Wei Zi*
Common English Name: Schisandra
Fruit
Part of Plant Used: Fruit
Nature: Warm
Taste: Sour (Schisandra is called the five-flavor fruit, and may actually be considered to have all five tastes.)

Meridians Entered: Lungs, Kidneys .
Common Usages: This herb is used in formulas to treat asthma with cough, shallow breathing and wheezing, frequent urination, early-morning diarrhea, spontaneous sweating and night sweats, insomnia, diabetes syndrome, and palpitations.
Traditional Usages and Functions: Contains leakage of Lung Qi and stops coughing; restrains Essence and stops diarrhea; stops excessive sweating; calms Spirit. This herb is used in formulas that support the Organs in their proper function, especially Kidneys and Liver, by restraining leakage of vital energy and Fluids.
Common Formulas Used In: Cerebral Tonic Pills; Concha Marguerita and Ligustrum; Eight Immortal Long Life Pill; Fritillaria Extract Tablet; Ginseng and Zizyphus; Xanthium and Magnolia.
Cautions in Use: Do not use where there are excess heat imbalances or in early stages of coughing.

125. Schizonepeta
荆芥

Latin Plant Name: Schizonepetae Tenu-foliae
Pinyin Mandarin Name: *Jing Jie*
Common English Name: Schizonepeta
Part of Plant Used: Stems and buds
Nature: Slightly warm
Taste: Acrid, aromatic
Meridians Entered: Lungs, Liver
Common Usages: This herb is used in formulas to treat symptoms of colds, flus, headache, skin eruptions, boils, itching, chills, fever, sore throat, bloody nose, vomiting blood, hemorrhoids, and spotting (bleeding) between menstrual periods (*OM: early stages of wind invasion*).
Traditional Usages and Functions: Releases Exterior and expels wind; encourages rash to surface and alleviates itching; stops bleeding.
Common Formulas Used In: Cnidium and Tea; Lonicera and Forsythia; Xanthium and Magnolia.
Cautions in Use: Do not use where there are Liver wind imbalances or where there are fully erupted sores.

126. Scirpus
三棱

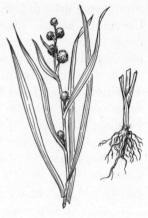

Latin Plant Name: Sparganii
Pinyin Mandarin Name: *San Leng*
Common English Name: Scirpus
Part of Plant Used: Root
Nature: Neutral
Taste: Bitter, acrid
Meridians Entered: Liver, Spleen
Common Usages: This herb is used in
formulas to treat pain and swelling in the
chest and abdominal area with symptoms
such as menstrual irregularity or absence, abdominal pain after child-
birth, and abdominal masses that are not malignant.
Traditional Usages and Functions: Forcefully breaks up congealed
Blood, moves Qi and alleviates pain; dissolves accumulations.
Common Formulas Used In: None in this book. Scirpus is commonly
found in stone-expelling and worm-eliminating formulas.
Cautions in Use: Do not use during pregnancy. Use with caution
where there are deficiency conditions.

127. Scrophularia
玄参

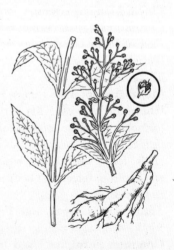

Latin Plant Name: Scrophulariae
Ningpoensis
Pinyin Mandarin Name: *Xuan Shen*
Common English Name: Scrophu-
laria
Part of Plant Used: Root
Nature: Cold
Taste: Salty, slightly bitter
Meridians Entered: Lungs, Stomach,
Kidneys
Common Usages: This herb is used
in formulas to treat symptoms such as constipation, dizziness, and
irritability after a feverish imbalance; swollen eyes and extremely sore
and swollen throat, bleeding due to heat and toxicity, boils, goiter,

thirst, and dry cough with thin phlegm *(OM: deficient Yin and fire conditions)*.

Traditional Usages and Functions: Clears heat and cools Blood; nourishes Yin; quells fire and detoxifies fire poison; softens hardness and dissipates nodules.

Common Formulas Used In: Ginseng and Zizyphus.

Cautions in Use: Use with caution where there is dampness of Spleen or Stomach, or where there is deficient Spleen diarrhea.

128. Scutellaria

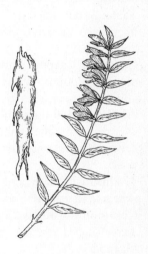

Latin Plant Name: Scutellariae Baiclaensis
Pinyin Mandarin Name: *Huang Qin*
Common English Name: Scute
Part of Plant Used: Root
Nature: Cold
Taste: Bitter
Meridians Entered: Heart, Lungs, Gall-bladder, Large Intestine
Common Usages: This herb is used in formulas to treat symptoms of red eyes, cough with shortness of breath, irritability, high blood pressure, headache, thick and yellow sputum, and diarrhea with fever and thirst; also used to treat nervousness, insomnia, and skin problems *(OM: internal-heat and damp-heat conditions)*.

Traditional Usages and Functions: Clears heat and quells fire, particularly in Upper Burner; drains damp heat; clears heat and calms the fetus; subdues ascending Liver Yang; harmonizes function between Liver and Spleen by treating Gallbladder.

Common Formulas Used In: Bupleurum and Dragon Bone; Cimicafuga; Gentiana; Minor Bupleurum; Prunella and Scutellaria; Qiang-Huo and Turmeric; Rhubarb and Scutellaria; Tang Gui and Gardenia.

Cautions in Use: Do not use where there is deficient Heat in Lungs, cold diarrhea or other conditions of cold in Middle Burner, or cold in Blood.

129. Siler
防風

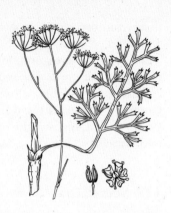

Latin Plant Name: Ledebouriellae Sesloidis
Pinyin Mandarin Name: *Fang Feng*
Common English Name: Siler
Part of Plant Used: Root
Nature: Slightly warm
Taste: Acrid, sweet
Meridians Entered: Bladder, Liver, Spleen
Common Usages: This herb is used in formulas to treat symptoms of skin eruptions, headache, chills, and body aches; swollen and achy joints and muscles with wandering joint pain; painful diarrhea and bright blood in the stools; and trembling of hands and feet and lockjaw symptoms when combined with specific other herbs *(OM: exterior wind symptoms; wind-damp symptoms; Intestinal wind symptoms; exterior wind).*
Traditional Usages and Functions: Releases exterior and expels wind; expels wind dampness and alleviates pain; expels wind.
Common Formulas Used In: Clematis and Stephania; Cnidium and Tea; Qiang-Huo and Turmeric; Tu-Huo and Loranthus; Xanthium and Magnolia.
Cautions in Use: Do not use where there is deficient Blood with spasms or deficient Yin with heat signs.

130. Soja Seed
淡豆豉

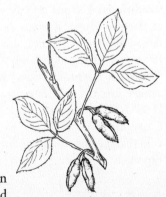

Latin Plant Name: Sojae Praeparatum
Pinyin Mandarin Name: *Dan Dou Chi*
Common English Name: Soja Seed
Part of Plant Used: Seed
Nature: Neutral
Taste: Sweet, slightly bitter
Meridians Entered: Lungs, Spleen
Common Usages: This herb is used in formulas to treat symptoms of colds and

flus with either fever or chills and chest tightness; also used to treat fevers accompanied by irritability, restlessness, and insomnia *(OM: exterior surface imbalances)*.

Traditional Usages and Functions: Releases exterior; alleviates irritability.

Common Formulas Used In: Lonicera and Forsythia.

Cautions in Use: Do not use where there is deficient Blood with spasms or deficient Yin with heat signs.

131. Sophora
槐花米

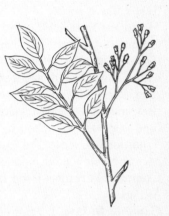

Latin Plant Name: Sophora Japonicae Immaturus

Pinyin Mandarin Name: *Huai Hua Mi*

Common English Name: Sophora

Part of Plant Used: Flower

Nature: Cool

Taste: Bitter

Meridians Entered: Liver, Large Intestine

Common Usages: This herb is used in formulas to treat bleeding hemorrhoids, coughing up of blood, nosebleeds, and uterine bleeding *(OM: damp-heat conditions; damp heat in Large Intestine);* also used to treat intestinal ulceration, headache, high blood pressure, red eyes, and dizziness *(OM: Liver heat)*.

Traditional Usages and Functions: Cools Blood and stops bleeding; cools Liver.

Common Formulas Used In: Prunella and Scutellaria.

Cautions in Use: Use with caution where there is a cold deficiency in Spleen or Stomach.

132. Stephania

漢防己

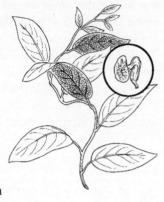

Latin Plant Name: Stephania Tetrandrae
Pinyin Mandarin Name: *Han Fang Ji*
Common English Name: Stephania
Part of Plant Used: Root
Nature: Cold
Taste: Bitter, acrid
Meridians Entered: Lungs, Spleen
Common Usages: This herb is used in formulas to treat inflammation of knees with spasms of hands and feet; gurgling intestines with bloating; edema of lower half of body with swollen legs and feet; arthritis and rheumatism; and high blood pressure *(OM: external damp-heat conditions)*. Also used as a diuretic.
Traditional Usages and Functions: Promotes urination and reduces edema; expels wind dampness and alleviates pain.
Common Formulas Used In: Clematis and Stephania; Stephania and Astragalus.
Cautions in Use: Do not use where there is internal dampness. Use cautiously with Yin deficiency.

133. Talc

滑石

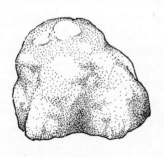

Latin Plant Name: Talcum
Pinyin Mandarin Name: *Hua Shi*
Common English Name: Talcum
Part of Plant Used: Whole mineral
Nature: Cold
Taste: Sweet, bland
Meridians Entered: Stomach, Bladder
Common Usages: This herb is used in formulas to treat painful, concentrated dark urination with associated symptoms of blood in urine; also used to treat fever, irritability, and thirst due to food poisoning or heatstroke *(OM: heat imbalances)*; also has been found useful in treating

small stones. May be used topically to treat some skin rashes *(OM: dampness)*.

Traditional Usages and Functions: Promotes urination and drains heat from Bladder; clears heat and releases summer heat; absorbs dampness; expels damp heat through the urine.

Common Formulas Used In: Dianthus.

Cautions in Use: Use cautiously during pregnancy. Do not use where there is deficient Spleen or sperm leakage, or where there are depleted fluids due to lengthy fevers or excessive urination.

134. Tribuli

白蒺藜

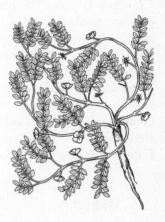

Latin Plant Name: Tribuli Terrestris

Pinyin Mandarin Name: *Bai Ji Li;* also *Ci Ji Li* and *Ji Li*

Common English Name: Tribulus

Part of Plant Used: Fruit

Nature: Warm

Taste: Acrid, bitter

Meridians Entered: Liver, Lungs

Common Usages: This herb is used in formulas to treat headaches, eye problems such as itching, conjunctivitis and weak vision, and nervousness; also used to treat high blood pressure *(OM: due to Liver Yang rising);* and rib pain *(OM: due to constrained Liver Qi [stress]).*

Traditional Usages and Functions: Extinguishes wind, alleviates pain, and brightens the eyes; extinguishes exterior wind; facilitates smooth flow of Liver Qi.

Common Formulas Used In: Rehmannia and Dogwood Fruit.

Cautions in Use: Use cautiously during pregnancy, or where there is deficient Qi or Blood.

135. Uncaria
鉤籐

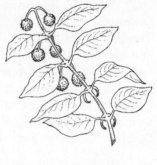

Latin Plant Name: Uncariae Cum Uncis
Pinyin Mandarin Name: *Gou Teng*
Common English Name: Gambir
Part of Plant Used: Stems and thorns
Nature: Cool
Taste: Sweet
Meridians Entered: Liver, Heart
Common Usages: This herb is used in formulas that treat high blood pressure, headaches, red eyes, irritability and dizziness *(OM: Liver Yang rising)*; also has been found useful in treating tremors, seizures, and Blood toxicity during pregnancy or childbirth *(OM: Liver heat with internal Liver wind)*.
Traditional Usages and Functions: Extinguishes wind and alleviates spasms; quells heat and pacifies Liver; releases exterior.
Common Formulas Used In: Leonuris and Achyranthes.
Remarks: When preparing as a tea, add Uncaria last.
Cautions in Use: None.

136. Walnut
胡桃仁

Latin Plant Name: Juglandis Regiae
Pinyin Mandarin Name: *Hu Tao Ren*
Common English Name: Walnut
Part of Plant Used: Meat of nut
Nature: Warm
Taste: Sweet
Meridians Entered: Kidneys, Lungs
Common Usages: This herb is used in formulas to treat cold and painful back and knees, impotence, insomnia, poor memory, kidney stones, leakage of sperm, and frequent urination; also used to treat weak coughs and wheezing *(OM: deficient Lungs and Kidneys)*; and constipation with over-all weakened condition such as found in the elderly or following a fever-ish disease.
Traditional Usages and Functions: Tonifies Kidneys and strengthens

back and knees; warms and holds in Lung Qi and helps Kidneys "grasp" Qi; moistens Intestines and moves stool.

Common Formulas Used In: Cerebral Tonic Pills.

Cautions in Use: Do not use where there are phlegm fire symptoms, hot cough, deficienct Yin with heat signs, or watery stools.

137. Xanthium

蒼耳子

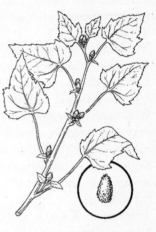

Latin Plant Name: Xanthii
Pinyin Mandarin Name: *Can Er Zi*
Common English Name: Cocklebur Fruit
Part of Plant Used: Fruit
Nature: Warm
Taste: Sweet, slightly bitter, poisonous
Meridians Entered: Liver, Lungs
Common Usages: This herb is used in formulas to treat headaches, sinus discharge and pain, arthritis with numbness, skin disorders, itching, and lumbago *(OM: due to dampness and wind);* also used to treat acute pain of headache and neck stiffness *(OM: due to wind).*

Traditional Usages and Functions: Opens nasal passages; disperses wind and expels dampness; Expels exterior wind.

Common Formulas Used In: Xanthium and Magnolia.

Cautions in Use: Do not use when headache or arthritis is due to deficient Blood.

138. Ziziphi Fruit

大棗

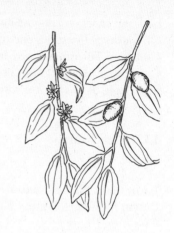

Latin Plant Name: Ziziphi Jujubae
Pinyin Mandarin Name: *Da Zao*
Common English Name: Red Date
Part of Plant Used: Fruit
Nature: Neutral
Taste: Sweet
Meridians Entered: Spleen, Stomach
Common Usages: This herb is used in
formulas for its nourishing, moisten-
ing, invigorating, and soothing effects.
It is used to treat insomnia, hysteria,
nervous imbalances, weak digestion, anemia, and fatigue from poor
metabolism; also used to help heal bruising and to enhance recovery
from illness. This herb increases circulation of other herbs in blood-
stream and moderates effects of stimulant herbs in people with weak
constitutions.

Traditional Usages and Functions: Tonifies Spleen and benefits
Stomach; nourishes Nutritive Qi, moistens dryness, and calms Spirit;
moderates and harmonizes other herbs.

Common Formulas Used In: Angelica; Bupleurum and Dragon
Bone; Ginseng and Astragalus; Ginseng and Longan; Major Six Herbs;
Minor Bupleurum; Pueraria Combination; Qiang-Huo and Turmeric;
Stephania and Astragalus.

Cautions in Use: Do not use where there are parasites, or where
there is dampness with signs of bloating or a sensation of fullness in
the upper abdomen. Use cautiously where there are damp phlegm
imbalances.

139. Ziziphi Seed
酸棗仁

Latin Plant Name: Ziziphi Spinosae
Pinyin Mandarin Name: *Suan Zao Ren*
Common English Name: Sour Date
Seed
Part of Plant Used: Seed
Nature: Neutral
Taste: Sweet, sour
Meridians Entered: Heart, Spleen,
Gallbladder
Common Usages: This herb is used in
formulas to treat irritability, insomnia,
palpitations, cold sweats, night sweats, spontaneous sweats, forgetful-
ness, amnesia, fright, and general weakness—especially due to long-
term stress.
Traditional Usages and Functions: Nourishes Heart and Liver and
calms Spirit; prevents abnormal sweating. Ziziphi seed is a nourishing
sedative that supports the nervous system and reduces leakages that
might weaken it.
Common Formulas Used In: Cerebral Tonic Pills; Ginseng and Longan; Ginseng and Zizyphus.
Cautions in Use: Use with caution where there is severe diarrhea or
excess heat.

CHAPTER SIX

Using Chinese Herbal Formulas: Introduction to 55 Healing Herbal Formulas

Herbal formulas provide the basis for treatment in herbal medicine. As we have already learned, they are made from the skillful and precise combination of single herbs, each of which plays a unique role in the formula. The primary herbs target a particular ailment or imbalance; the secondary herbs synergistically interact with them to enhance their healing effect, to nourish and strengthen the individual's overall health, and to offset any unwanted effects. In addition, formulas can be adapted, by adding or subtracting specific herbs, or by adjusting dosages, to match an individual's special health needs. Again, we encourage you to work with a traditional Oriental Medicine practitioner when you begin using herbal formulas.

How Formulas Are Dispensed and Used

Herbal formulas are usually prescribed, and frequently dispensed, by the practitioner. Alternatively, the patient may be given a formula "prescription" by the practitioner and then referred to a herbal pharmacist or supplier. Herbal pharmacists and suppliers (listed in the appendix) either provide herbal formulations in standard patent forms, or they weigh, blend, and package the raw herbs for the patient so that the herbs may be made into a tea or broth at home.

Patent Formulas

Many formulas—and almost all those listed in Chapter Seven—are already available in what are called *patent* forms. These premixed standard herbal formulations are prepared and sold by herbal pharmacists and herbal suppliers, in a variety of forms:

- *Pills, Tablets, and/or Capsules* taken orally at specific times throughout the day.
- *Powders and/or Granules* made into a tea or broth by adding boiling water and then drunk a cup at a time throughout the day.
- *Oils, Liniments, Creams, and Plasters* applied externally to skin wounds, rashes, fractures, and inflammations.
- *Tinctures or Liqueurs* (liquid formulations of herbs steeped in wine or another form of alcohol) drunk as fortifying tonics during the day. (The alcohol content may be evaporated before drinking by adding an equal amount of boiling water to the tincture and allowing it to steep for a few minutes.)
- *Herbal Porridges* (teas or herbal granular formulations mixed in a base of rice and/or millet) cooked on the stovetop like oatmeal and then eaten as a breakfast cereal (or as a snack throughout the day).

Either your practitioner, the pharmacist, or the instructions that come with the patent medication itself will provide you with dosage information.

Teas

You may also make your own medicinal teas from the herbal formulas provided in Chapter Seven. The herb quantities, given in grams in this book, will make a one day's supply of tea. Prepare only one day's supply at a time. (If your practitioner has not given you prepackaged daily supplies of the formulation, have the herbal pharmacist or supplier weigh, blend, prepackage, and label the herbs for you. Then store the herbs in a cool dry place until you are ready to use them.)

To prepare an herbal tea:

- In a large glass, ceramic, or stainless-steel pot with lid, add two quarts of pure spring or distilled water and the herbs.

- Bring the mixture to a boil, then lower heat, cover the pot, and simmer for twenty to forty minutes—until herbal mixture is about one half its original volume. If you are using any aromatic herbs in your formula (and they are noted in the herb entries), add them to the pot during the last five minutes of cooking.
- Remove mixture from heat and strain the liquid through a stainless-steel sieve (a tea strainer also works well) into a clean bowl, jar, or pitcher; reserve and set aside liquid.
- Place the herb dregs back into the pot and add 1 fresh quart of pure spring or distilled water.
- Bring the mixture to a boil again, then lower heat, cover the pot, and simmer for about twenty minutes, or until liquid is reduced to about three cups (twenty-four ounces).
- Remove mixture from heat and again strain through a stainless-steel sieve, adding the new liquid to the first reserved batch. You should have about one and a half to two quarts of tea. Discard the herb dregs, or add them to your compost pile. The tea may be stored in the refrigerator.
- Drink a large cup of the herbal tea, warm, three times a day on an empty stomach, one half hour before meals. Before a scheduled dose, remove the tea from the refrigerator and let it stand at room temperature for about one half hour. Then briefly warm the tea on the stovetop or by adding a few teaspoons of boiling water. Never microwave an herbal tea.

The fifty-five formulas described in Chapter Seven are among the finest, and most famous, in Oriental Medicine's healing pharmacopoeia. Almost all are available in patent forms, and thus they are readily obtainable from traditional practitioners, herbal pharmacists, and/or herbal suppliers.

The formulas are listed numerically in alphabetical order by their most common English or Chinese name.

The common symptoms for which the formula is most frequently prescribed are described in conventional medical terms under "Common Usages."

The traditional symptoms for which the formula is most often prescribed, together with the formula's therapeutic effects in the body, are described in the language of Oriental Medicine under "Traditional Usages and Functions."

The English transliteration and pinyin Mandarin names of the formula are also provided, together with the Chinese ideogram for the formula. As with the single herbs, the Chinese ideograms can be quite helpful for identification purposes if you are buying your formulas from a neighborhood supplier. The forms in which the formula is available— or may be used, as in the case of teas—are also given under "Forms Used."

The ingredients of each formula are listed by their pinyin Mandarin and common English or Latin names, together with a brief description of the herb's healing action (under "Traditional Herb Function"). The part of the herb commonly used in a particular formula is also indicated in abbreviated form (e.g., *rt.* for *root*; see key below), after its English or Latin name. With two or three exceptions, almost all the herbs used in these formulas are also listed in Chapter Five, so you may refer back to that chapter for more information on any one herb. The quantities needed for a one day's supply of herbal tea are also provided in grams for each herb.

Finally, any contraindications or cautions about a formula's use are listed under "Cautions in Use."

ABBREVIATION KEY TO PART OF PLANT USED IN FORMULA:

bk.	=	bark
cx. rx.	=	cross section of radix
fl.	=	flower
fr.	=	fruit
hb.	=	whole plant
imm. fl.	=	immature flower
imm. fr.	=	immature fruit
pl.	=	peel
rhz.	=	rhizome
rt.	=	root
rx.	=	radix
sd.	=	seed

CHAPTER SEVEN

An Herbal Medicine Chest: 55 Healing Herbal Formulas

1. Agastache Formula 藿香正氣丸

Common Usages: For the symptoms of stomach flu. Also used for other gastrointestinal disturbances with accompanying symptoms of headache, fever, nausea, vomiting, chills, diarrhea, fullness in chest, abdominal pain, and/or intestinal noise.

Traditional Usages and Functions: Used to tonify Spleen and harmonize Stomach. Clears heat and dispels chill.

English Transliteration: Agastache Formula

Pinyin Mandarin Name: *Huo Shang Zheng Qi Wan*

Forms Used: May be made into a tea or used in patent or granular forms.

Pinyin Name	Common English Name	Quantity in grams	Traditional Herb Function
Huo xiang	Agastache, hb.	1.0-3.0	Releases exterior; expels wind; harmonizes Middle Burner
Zi su ye	Perilla, fr.	1.0	Releases exterior; expels wind; harmonizes Middle Burner

Pinyin Name	Common English Name	Quantity in grams	Traditional Herb Function
Bai zhi	Angelica, rt.	1.0-1.5	Expels wind; opens nasal passages
Fu ling	Poria (fungus)	1.0-3.0	Drains Spleen dampness
Ban xia	Pinellia, rhz.	2.0-5.0	Drys damp; transforms phlegm; calms Stomach
Chen pi	Citrus, pl. (aged)	2.0	Moves Qi; strengthens Stomach; stops vomiting
Gan cao	Licorice, rx.	1.5	Moistens Lungs; stops coughing; harmonizes other herbs
Sheng jiang	Ginger, fresh rhz.	1.0	Disperses cold; adjusts Nutritive Qi
Bai zhu	Atractylodes, rhz.	2.0-3.0	Tonifies Spleen Qi; dries dampness
Hou po	Magnolia, bk.	2.0	Moves Qi and dampness; directs rebellious Qi downward
Da fu pi	Areca, husk	1.0	Moves Qi; expels damp
Jie geng	Platycodon, rt.	2.0	Circulates Lung Qi; soothes diaphragm

Cautions in Use: None.

2. Anemarrhena, Phellodendron, and Rehmannia Formula 知柏地黄丸

Common Usages: For menopausal hot flashes; night sweats; hot palms and soles; lower-back pain; insomnia; chronic sore throat; and chronic bladder infections.

Traditional Usages and Functions: Used for heat imbalances due to deficiency of Kidney yin, and for dampness in lower third of body due to yin deficiency. Nourishes Kidneys and clears heat.

English Transliteration: Anemarrhena, Phellodendron, and Rehmannia Formula

Pinyin Mandarin Name: *Zhi Bai Di Huang Wan*

Forms Used: May be made into a tea or used in patent or granular forms.

Pinyin Name	Common English Name	Quantity in grams	Traditional Herb Function
Shu di huang	Rehmannia (steamed)	4.0	Tonifies Liver and Kidneys; nourishes yin
Ze xie	Alisma, rhz.	3.0	Purges fire; helps Rehmannia
Shan zhu yu	Cornus Officinalis, fr.	3.0-4.5	Nourishes Liver; astringes essence
Mu dan pi	Moutan, cx. rx.	3.0	Drains Liver fire; cools Blood
Shan yao	Dioscoria, rx.	3.0-4.5	Tonifies Spleen Qi
Fu ling	Poria (fungus)	3.0	Strengthens Spleen; moves dampness
Huang bai	Phellodendron, bark	1.5-2.0	Drains damp heat; quells Kidney fire
Zhi mu	Anemarrhena, rhz.	1.5-2.0	Nourishes yin; moistens dry, clear heat

Cautions in Use: None.

3. Angelica Formula   當 歸 片

Common Usages: For chronic blood deficiencies and for blood loss after surgery, childbirth, or trauma. Also used for menstrual cramps, strengthening fingernails, fatigue, and weakness.

Traditional Usages and Functions: Used for Qi and Blood deficiencies, including Blood heat and stagnation. Nourishes Blood; fortifies Qi; tonifies Spleen Qi.

English Transliteration: Angelica Formula

Pinyin Mandarin Name: *Tang Gui Pian*

Forms Used: May be made into a tea or used in patent form.

Pinyin Name	Common English Name	Quantity in grams	Traditional Herb Function
Tang gui	Angelica, rt.	7.0	Tonifies and invigorates Blood
Chuan xiang	Ligusticum, rhz.	1.0	Invigorates Blood; moves Qi
Bai zhu	Atractylodes, rhz.	1.0	Tonifies Spleen Qi; drys dampness
Da zao	Ziziphi, fr.	1.0	Tonifies Spleen; benefits Stomach

Cautions in Use: None.

4. Apricot Seed and Fritillaria Formula

三蛇胆川贝液

Common Usages: For coughs with thick and stubborn yellow or green phlegm. Also combined with other formulas that treat bronchitis, asthma, and similar respiratory imbalances.

Traditional Usages and Functions: Resolves phlegm; clears heat; stops cough.

English Transliteration: Apricot Seed and Fritillaria Formula

Pinyin Mandarin Name: *San She Dan Chuan Bei Ye*

Forms Used: May be used in patent form.

Pinyin Name	Common English Name	Quantity in grams	Traditional Herb Function
Chuan bei mu	Fritillaria, bulb	5.0	Clears heat; transforms phlegm
Xing ren	Apricot, sd.	4.0	Relieves cough; stops wheezing
San she dan	Snake Gall Trio	1.0	Clears heat; transforms phlegm

NOTE: This formula is available only in ampules as a liquid extract. As such, it is the only formula in the book available only as a patent formula.

Cautions in Use: None.

5. Apricot Seed and Linum Formula

麻子仁丸

Common Usages: For chronic constipation, often accompanied by hemorrhoids, as frequently seen in the elderly. Also used for the acute constipation that sometimes occurs after long periods of inactivity or during travel.

Traditional Usages and Functions: Used for intestinal dryness with heat, accompanied by symptoms of sparse body fluids, hard and dry stools, and frequent urination. Moistens Intestines and promotes bowel movements.

English Transliteration: Apricot Seed and Linum Formula

Pinyin Mandarin Name: *Ma Zi Ren Wan*

Forms Used: May be made into a tea or used in patent or granular forms.

Pinyin Name	Common English Name	Quantity in grams	Traditional Herb Function
Da huang	Rhubarb, rhz.	4.0	Drains heat; moves stool
Zhi shi	Aurantium, imm. fr.	2.0	Breaks up stagnant Qi; moves stool
Hou po	Magnolia, bk.	2.0	Moves Qi and dampness; directs rebellious Qi downward
Huo ma ren	Linum, sd.	5.0	Nourishes and moistens the Intestines
Xing ren	Apricot, sd.	5.0	Relieves coughs; stops wheezing
Bai shao	Peony Alba, rx.	3.0	Pacifies Liver; tonifies Blood; preserves yin

Cautions in Use: None. This is a mild, demulcent laxative that is unlikely to cause the dependency that some other laxatives do. Do not use while pregnant.

6. Bupleurum and Dragon Bone Formula 柴 胡 加 龍 骨 牡 蠣 湯

Common Usages: For anxiety, insomnia, irritability, emotional instability, palpitations, delirium, fatigue, constipation, high blood pressure, palpitations in abdomen (above navel), and nervous spasm. Also used for symptoms associated with drug withdrawal.

Traditional Usages and Functions: Harmonizes interior and exterior; pacifies the spirit.

English Transliteration: Bupleurum and Dragon Bone Formula

Pinyin Mandarin Name: *Chai Hu Jia Long Gu Mu Li Tang*

Forms Used: May be made into a tea or used in granular form.

Pinyin Name	Common English Name	Quantity in grams	Traditional Herb Function
Chai hu	Bupleurum, rt.	5.0	Relaxes constrained Liver Qi
Huang qin	Scutellaria, rx.	2.5	Clears heat; drains damp heat
Long gu	Dragon Bone	2.5	Settles and calms the spirit; pacifies Liver
Mu li	Oyster Shell	2.5	Benefits yin; settles and calms the spirit

Pinyin Name	Common English Name	Quantity in grams	Traditional Herb Function
Gui zhi	Cinnamon, twig	3.0	Warms channels; strengthens Heart yang
Fu ling	Poria (fungus)	3.0	Quiets Heart; calms spirit; transforms phlegm
Ban xia	Pinellia, rhz.	4.0	Drys damp; transforms phlegm; calms Stomach
Sheng jiang	Ginger, fresh rhz.	2.5	Disperses cold; adjusts Nutritive Qi
Da huang	Rhubarb, rhz.	1.0	Drains damp heat and excess heat from Blood
Ren shen	Ginseng, rx.	2.5	Benefits Heart Qi; calms spirit
Da zao	Ziziphi, fr.	2.5	Tonifies Spleen; benefits Stomach

Cautions in Use: Not to be used during pregnancy. Do not use when there is a tendency to diarrhea. Avoid use at the onset of cold or flu, but can be used once recovery has begun.

7. Bupleurum, Inula, and Cyperus Formula 舒肝丸

Common Usages: For stress-related gastrointestinal symptoms including bloating and fullness in the upper abdomen, poor appetite, heartburn, belching, and vomiting with cold limbs and facial flushing. May also be used for chronic hepatitis, simple hiatal hernia, gastritis, gastroduodenal ulcer, and gastric pain.

Traditional Usages and Functions: Used for stagnant Liver Qi, rebellious Stomach Qi, and for hysteria related to Liver and Qi stagnation. Soothes Liver, regulates Qi and Blood, and relieves pain.

English Transliteration: Bupleurum and Evodia

Pinyin Mandarin Name: *Shu Gan Wan*

Forms Used: May be made into a tea or used in patent or granular forms.

Pinyin Name	Common English Name	Quantity in grams	Traditional Herb Function
Chai hu	Bupleurum, rt.	2.0	Smoothes Liver; relieves stress
Bai shao	Peony Alba, rx.	3.0	Nourishes Blood; pacifies Liver

Pinyin Name	Common English Name	Quantity in grams	Traditional Herb Function
Chen pi	Citrus, pl. (aged)	2.0	Moves Qi; strengthens Stomach; stops vomiting
Xiang fu	Cyperus, rt.	3.0	Resolves Liver Qi; relieves pain
Zhi ke	Auranti, fr.	2.0	Moves Qi; reduces sensation of pressure
Hou po	Magnolia, bk.	2.0	Moves Qi and dampness; directs rebellious Qi downward
Sha ren	Cardamon, sd.	2.0	Moves Qi; strengthens Stomach
Qing pi	Citri Immaturi	3.0	Moves Liver Qi and accumulations
Yan hu suo	Corydalis, rhz.	3.0	Moves Blood and Qi; alleviates pain
Mu dan pi	Moutan, cx. rx.	3.0	Drains Liver fire; cools Blood
Xuan fu hua	Inula, fl.	1.5	Directs Qi downward
Fo shou	Citron, Finger Fructus	1.5	Moves Qi; alleviates pain
Gan cao	Licorice, rx.	1.5	Tonifies Spleen; benefits Qi
Jiang huang	Curcuma, rhz.	1.5	Moves Qi; alleviates pain
Chen xiang	Aquilaria, wood	1.0	Moves Qi; alleviates pain
Bai dou kou	Cardamom, sd., inf.	1.0	Moves Qi; transforms stagnation and dampness
Tan xiang	Sandalwood	1.0	Moves Qi; alleviates pain

Cautions in Use: None.

8. Bupleurum and Tang Gui Formula   逍 遙 丸

Common Usages: For all types of stress-related problems, especially female depression with blood deficiency, bloating, poor appetite, dry throat, heaviness in the head, and/or bitter taste in the mouth. Frequently used for menstrual and menopausal difficulties. Also used for chronic liver problems where there is no jaundice.

Traditional Usages and Functions: Smoothes Liver Qi, strengthens Spleen, nourishes Blood, and restores harmony between Spleen and Stomach.
English Transliteration: Bupleurum and Tang Gui
Pinyin Mandarin Name: *Xiao Yao Wan*
Forms Used: May be made into a tea or used in patent or granular forms.

Pinyin Name	Common English Name	Quantity in grams	Traditional Herb Function
Chai hu	Bupleurum, rt.	3.0	Smoothes Liver; relieves stress
Tang gui	Angelica, rt.	3.0	Tonifies Liver; harmonizes Blood
Bai shao	Peony Alba, rx.	3.0	Nourishes Blood; pacifies Liver
Bai zhu	Atractylodes, rhz.	3.0	Tonifies Spleen; benefits Qi
Fu ling	Poria (fungus)	3.0	Strengthens Spleen; harmonizes Middle Burner
Bo he	Peppermint, leaf	1.0	Allows Liver Qi to flow
Gan cao	Licorice, rx.	1.5	Tonifies Spleen; benefits Qi
Sheng jiang pi	Ginger, fresh rhz.	2.0	Disperses cold; adjusts Nutritive Qi

Cautions in Use: Formula sometimes requires adjustment by the practitioner.

9. Cerebral Tonic Pills 補 腦 丸

Common Usages: To enhance brain function and to treat the symptoms of poor concentration and memory associated with arteriosclerotic conditions such as Alzheimer's. May also be used for restlessness, mental agitation, fatigue, and insomnia.
Traditional Usages and Functions: For internal dampness that interferes with clarity of thought. Nourishes Heart yin, clears Heart phlegm, nourishes Brain, and calms spirit. Also has been used to treat manic episodes and seizures associated with Liver-Blood deficiency and internal wind.

English Transliteration: Schisandra and Zizyphus Formula
Pinyin Mandarin Name: *Bu Nao Wan*
Forms Used: May be made into a tea or used in patent form. This
formula works best when Ginko Biloba extract is also taken.

Pinyin Name	Common English Name	Quantity in grams	Traditional Herb Function
Wu wei zi	Schisandra, fr.	6.0	Strengthens Kidney and Heart Qi; calms spirit; improves sleep and memory
Suan zao ren	Ziziphi, sd.	4.5	Nourishes Heart and Liver; calms spirit
Tang gui	Angelica, rt.	3.0	Tonifies and invigorates Blood
Rou cong rong	Cistanches, stem	2.5	Tonifies Kidneys; strengthens yang
Gou qi zi	Lycium, fr.	2.5	Nourishes Kidney and Liver yin; benefits essence
Hu tao ren	Walnut	2.5	Tonifies Kidneys; benefits brain
Bai zi ren	Biota, sd.	2.0	Nourishes Heart; calms spirit
Chang pu	Acorus, rhz.	2.0	Opens orifices; vaporizes phlegm
Tian nan xing	Arisaema, tubers	2.0	Dries dampness; expels phlegm
Hu po	Amber, resin	2.0	Sedates and calms spirit
Tian ma	Gastrodia, rhz.	2.0	Pacifies Liver; extinguishes wind
Long chi	Dragon Teeth	2.0	Settles and calms spirit; helps sleep
Yuan zhi	Polygala	2.0	Calms spirit; expels phlegm

Cautions in Use: Excessive use may lead to Spleen and Stomach Qi
disturbances that are manifested as indigestion and poor appetite.

10. Cimicafuga Formula 乙字湯

Common Usages: For hemorrhoids accompanied by chronic constipation, local pain, and bleeding. Also used for prolapse of the rectum; and for varicose veins concurrent with hemorrhoids.

Traditional Usages and Functions: Clears heat; relieves hemorrhoids; promotes bowel movements.

English Transliteration: Cimicafuga Formula

Pinyin Mandarin Name: *Yi Zi Tang*

Forms Used: May be made into a tea or used in granular form.

Pinyin Name	Common English Name	Quantity in grams	Traditional Herb Function
Chai hu	Bupleurum, rt.	5.0	Raises yang Qi in presence of Spleen and Stomach deficiencies
Sheng ma	Cimicifuga, rt.	1.5	Raises yang Qi
Tang gui	Angelica, rt.	6.0	Tonifies and invigorates Blood; moistens stool
Gan cao	Licorice, rx.	2.0	Tonifies Spleen; benefits Qi, harmonizes other herbs
Huang qin	Scutellaria, rx.	3.0	Clears heat; drains damp heat
Da huang	Rhubarb, rhz.	1.0	Drains damp heat; detoxifies fire poison

Cautions in Use: Not to be used during pregnancy.

11. Citrus and Pinellia Formula 二陳丸

Common Usages: For coughs with profuse phlegm, accompanied by abdominal bloating, nausea, vomiting, dizziness, or Heart palpitations. Also used as a hangover remedy.

Traditional Uses and Functions: Regulates Qi, harmonizes Spleen and Stomach, and dispels congestions in Stomach, Lungs, or sinuses. Useful in treating general dampness or poor metabolism.

English Transliteration: Citrus and Pinellia

Pinyin Mandarin Name: *Er Chen Wan*

Forms Used: May be made into a tea or used in patent or granular forms.

Pinyin Name	Common English Name	Quantity in grams	Traditional Herb Function
Ban xia	Pinellia, rhz.	5.0	Dries damp; transforms phlegm; calms Stomach
Fu ling	Poria (fungus)	5.0	Strengthens Spleen; moves dampness
Chen pi	Citrus, pl. (aged)	4.0	Moves Qi; strengthens Stomach; melts phlegm
Gan cao	Licorice, rx.	1.0	Tonifies Spleen; benefits Qi
Sheng jiang pi	Ginger, Fresh rhz.	3.0	Disperses cold; adjusts Nutritive Qi

Cautions in Use: None.

12. Clematis and Stephania Formula　疏經活血湯

Common Usages: For gout, arthritis of the knees and ankles, sciatica, lower-back pain, some types of paralysis, high blood pressure, numbness and pain in the lower back and legs, and postpartum thrombosis. Clematis and Stephania is particularly good for elderly people who have a long history of prescription-drug use and/or a history of surgery that has impaired circulation and caused stagnant Blood conditions.

Traditional Usages and Functions: To treat symptoms of wind dampness and wind chill, especially below the waist. Unblocks and relaxes the channels and activates Blood; dispels wind and dampness.

English Transliteration: Clematis and Stephania

Pinyin Mandarin Name: *Shu Jing Huo Xue Tang*

Forms Used: May be made into a tea or used in patent or granular forms.

Pinyin Name	Common English Name	Quantity in grams	Traditional Herb Function
Tang gui	Angelica sinensis	2.0	Tonifies and invigorates Blood
Bai shao	Peony Alba, rx.	2.5	Pacifies Liver; tonifies Blood; preserves yin
Chuan xiang	Ligusticum, rhz.	2.0	Invigorates Blood; moves Qi
Sheng di huang	Rehmannia (raw)	2.0	Cools upward Heart fire; nourishes yin

Pinyin Name	Common English Name	Quantity in grams	Traditional Herb Function
Tao ren	Persica, sd. pit	2.0	Breaks up congealed Blood; moistens dryness
Fu ling	Poria Cocos (fungus)	2.0	Drains Spleen dampness
Bai zhu	Atractylodes Alba	2.0	Tonifies Spleen Qi; dries dampness
Chen pi	Citrus, pl. (aged)	1.5	Moves Qi, strengthens Stomach; stops vomiting
Qiang-huo	Notoptergi	1.5	Releases exterior; disperses cold and damp; penetrates obstruction; alleviates pain
Bai zhi	Angelica, rt.	1.0	Expels wind; opens nasal passages
Wei ling xian	Clematis, rt.	1.5	Expels wind damp; alleviates pain
Han fang ji	Stephania	1.5	Expels wind damp; promotes urination; reduces edema
Long dan cao	Gentiana Scabra	1.5	Drain Liver and Gall-bladder damp and fire
Fang feng	Siler	1.5	Expels wind damp; alleviates pain
Niu xi	Achyranthes	1.5	Strengthens sinews and bones; benefits joints
Sheng jiang	Ginger, fresh rhz.	1.5	Disperses cold; adjusts Nutritive Qi
Gan cao	Licorice, rx.	1.0	Moistens Lungs; stops coughing; harmonizes other herbs

Cautions in Use: Do not use during pregnancy.

13. Cnidium and Tea Formula　　川芎茶調散

Common Usages: For headaches, particularly sudden headaches, with associated symptoms of migraine, pain on top of head, chills, fever, dizziness, congestion, and/or sinusitis.

Traditional Usages and Functions: For wind-heat or wind-cold conditions. Dispels wind, clears heat, and relieves pain.

English Transliteration: Cnidium (Ligusticum) and Tea Formula
Pinyin Mandarin Name: *Chuan Qiong Cha Tiao Wan*
Forms Used: May be made into a tea or used in patent or granular forms.

Pinyin Name	Common English Name	Quantity in grams	Traditional Herb Function
Chuan xiang	Ligusticum, rhz.	4.0	Invigorates Blood; moves Qi; stops headache
Qiang-huo	Angelica sylvestris, rt. stalk	2.0	Releases exterior; disperses cold and damp; penetrates obstruction; alleviates pain
Fang feng	Siler, rt.	1.5	Expels wind dampness; alleviates pain
Jing jie	Schizonepeta, hb.	4.0	Releases exterior; expels wind
Bai zhi	Angelica, rx.	2.0	Expels wind; opens nasal passages
Xi xin	Asarum, hb.	1.0	Expels wind; disperses cold; alleviates pain
Bo he	Peppermint, leaf	8.0	Disperses wind heat; benefits throat
Cha ye	Green tea, camellia	3.0	Cools head; balances other herbs
Gan cao	Licorice, rx.	2.0	Harmonizes other herbs

Note: If preparing at home, do not cook for more than ten minutes. For raw herb formula prepared from scratch, a strong, brewed green tea is cooked separately and sipped separately. In granular and patent Cnidium and Tea formulas, green tea is included in the prepared form.

Cautions in Use: Do not use with Liver yang excess or Qi and Blood deficiency headaches.

14. Concha Marguerita and Ligustrum Formula 安神補心丸

Common Usages: Used frequently for anxiety and/or depression, and for the mental stress associated with overwork and accompanied by insomnia, dizziness, ringing in the ears, forgetfulness, and/or heart palpitations.

Traditional Usages and Functions: Tonifies Heart and Blood; calms Shen (spirit). Used for weakness of the Kidneys and Heart.

English Transliteration: Concha Marguerita and Ligustrum
Pinyin Mandarin Name: *An Shen Bu Xin Wan*
Forms Used: May be made into a tea or used in patent form.

Pinyin Name	Common English Name	Quantity in grams	Traditional Herb Function
Zhen zhu mu	Marguerite concha, shell	10.0	Pacifies Liver; calms spirit
Nu zhen zi	Ligustrum, fr.	2.5	Nourishes and tonifies Kidney and Liver yin
Han lian cao	Eclipta, hb.	2.0	Nourishes and tonifies Kidney and Liver yin
Dan shen	Salvia, rt.	2.0	Invigorates Blood; clears heat
He huan pi	Albizzia	2.0	Invigorates Blood; calms spirit
Tu si zi	Cuscuta, sd.	2.0	Tonifies Kidneys; benefits essence
Wu wei zi	Schisandra, fr.	1.0	Contains leakage of Lung Qi; calms spirit
Chang pu	Acorus, rhz.	1.0	Opens orifices; vaporizes phlegm
Sheng di huang	Rehmannia, rt. (raw)	1.0	Cools upward Heart fire; nourishes yin

Cautions in Use: Extended overuse of this formula may cause indigestion and poor appetite. Do not use this formula if there is a thick, greasy coat on tongue with poor digestion.

15. Corydalis Formula　　延 胡 索 芍 葯 甘 草 湯

Common Usages: For pain due to spasm and cramping and associated with menstruation, muscle spasms, smooth-muscle pains and intestinal cramping (colic), bronchial spasm, Bladder spasm and stones, and/or Gallbladder pain.
Traditional Usages and Functions: Moves Blood and Qi, softens Liver, relieves pain and spasms, and relaxes muscles. Not useful for pain due to wind invasion.
English Transliteration: Corydalis Formula
Pinyin Mandarin Name: Combination of *Shao Yao Gan Cao Tang* and *Yan Hu Suo*
Forms Used: May be used as a tea or in patent form.

Pinyin Name	Common English Name	Quantity in grams	Traditional Herb Function
Yan hu suo	Corydalis, rhz.	3.0	Moves Blood and Qi; alleviates pain
Bai shao	Peony Alba, rx.	3.0	Pacifies Liver; alleviates pain
Gan cao	Licorice, rx.	3.0	Tonifies Spleen; harmonizes other herbs; soothes spasm

Cautions in Use: Do not use this formula for Bladder or Gallbladder pain without also working with a practitioner who can monitor any complications that may arise.

16. Corydalis Tuber Formula 延 胡 索 止 痛 片

Common Usages: Used specifically for headache pain. May also be used for Stomach and Gallbladder pain, pain due to injury or rheumatism, menstrual cramping, sinus headaches, and joint inflammation.
Traditonal Usages and Function: Regulates Qi and Blood in channels; alleviates pain.
English Transliteration: Corydalis Tuber Formula
Pinyin Mandarin Name: *Yan Hu Suo Zhi Tong Pian*
Forms Used: May be made into a tea or used in patent or granular forms.

Pinyin Name	Common English Name	Quantity in grams	Traditional Herb Function
Yan hu suo	Corydalis, rhz.	3.0-5.0	Moves Blood and Qi; alleviates pain
Bai zhi	Angelica, rt.	1.0-1.5	Expels wind; opens nasal passages

Cautions in Use: Prohibited during pregnancy.

17. Cyperus and Ligusticum Formula 越 鞠 丸

Common Usages: To treat symptoms associated with irregular diet, exposure to excessive heat or cold, severe mood swings, and/or anxiety. Such symptoms may be manifested as a stifling sensation in chest and abdomen, back pain, shortness of breath, and/or coughing. Other symptoms may include abdominal distension, belching, acid reflux, hiatal hernia, irregular bowel habits, and menstrual imbalances.

Traditional Usages and Functions: Specifically to treat the condition known as "Plum Pit Qi"—the sensation of a plum pit stuck at the base of the throat—which is caused by constrained or stagnant Qi. Spleen and/or Liver constraint may also be present. Promotes movement of Qi and releases constraint.
English Transliteration: Escape Restraint Pill
Pinyin Mandarin Name: *Yue Ju Wan*
Forms Used: May be used as a tea, made into pills, or in patent form.

Pinyin Name	Common English Name	Quantity in grams	Traditional Herb Function
Cang zhu	Atractylodes, rhz.	8.0	Dries dampness; strengthens Spleen
Chuan xiang	Ligusticum, rhz.	8.0	Invigorates Blood; moves Qi
Xiang fu	Cyperus, rt.	8.0	Resolves Liver Qi; disperses Qi stagnation
Zhi zi	Gardenia, fr.	8.0	Drains damp heat; cools Blood
Shen qu	Massa Fermenta	8.0	Dissolves stagnation of food; harmonizes Stomach

Cautions in Use: None.

18. Dianthus Formula   八正散
Common Usages: Used for urinary-tract infections where there is dark, turbid urine, painful and difficult urination, urge to urinate frequently, thirst, dry throat, pain, fullness in lower abdomen, and tendency toward constipation; also used for yeast infections, herpetic, burning urination; postsurgical numbness and infection of urinary tract, and the urinary heat symptoms that may result from some birth-control medications. May also be used to treat gonorrhea and acute nephritis in conjunction with conventional treatment.
Traditional Usages and Functions: Clears heat, purges fire, and promotes water metabolism.
English Transliteration: Dianthus Formula
Pinyin Mandarin Name: *Ba Zheng San*
Forms Used: May be made into a tea or used in patent or granular forms.

Pinyin Name	Common English Name	Quantity in grams	Traditional Herb Function
Qu mai	Dianthus, hb.	3.0	Clears heat; promotes urination
Mu tong	Akebia, stem	3.0	Promotes urination; drains heat
Bian xu	Polygonum Avicularis	3.0	Promotes urination; clears damp heat
Che qian zi	Plantago, sd.	1.5	Promotes urination; clears heat
Deng xin cao	Juncus	2.0	Promotes urination; clears heat downward
Hua shi	Talc	5.0	Promotes urination; expels damp heat
Zhi zi	Gardenia, fr.	3.0	Drains damp heat in three Burners
Da huang	Rhubarb, rhz.	1.0	Drains damp heat; detoxifies fire poison
Gan cao	Licorice, rx.	1.5	Harmonizes other herbs

Cautions in Use: May cause loose stool in some people. Be careful using this formula if there is chronic diarrhea. Drink lots of water to avoid dehydration.

19. Eight Immortal Long Life Pill 八仙長壽丸

Common Usages: For coughs with dry throat. May also be used for hot flashes; sweating; chronic weakness with thirst; lower-back pain; and weak knees.

Traditional Usages and Functions: Used for deficiencies of Lung and Kidney yin, and yin-related Lung heat. Nourishes Lung and Kidney yin; moistens and cools Lungs.

English Transliteration: Rehmannia and Ophiopogon Combination

Pinyin Mandarin Name: *Ba Xian Chang Shou Wan*

Forms Used: May be made into a tea or used in patent formula.

Pinyin Name	Common English Name	Quantity in grams	Traditional Herb Function
Shu di huang	Rehmannia (steamed)	4.0	Tonifies Liver and Kidneys; nourishes yin
Ze xie	Alisma, rhz.	3.0	Purges fire; helps Rehmannia

Pinyin Name	Common English Name	Quantity in grams	Traditional Herb Function
Shan zhu yu	Cornus Officinalis, fr.	3.0-4.5	Nourishes Liver; astringes Essence
Mu dan pi	Moutan, cx. rx.	3.0	Drains Liver fire; cools Blood
Shan yao	Dioscoria, rx.	3.0-4.5	Tonifies Spleen Qi
Fu ling	Poria (fungus)	3.0	Strengthens Spleen; moves dampness
Mai men dong	Ophiopogon, rt.	3.0	Nourishes yin; moistens Lungs; stops cough
Wu wei zi	Schisandra, fr.	1.0	Contains leakage of Lung Qi; stops cough

Cautions in Use: Make sure that dampness is under control before using this formula for any extended period of time; discontinue use if headaches occur or if a thick coating develops on the tongue. To help with this, try to avoid greasy foods and excessive dairy products when using this formula.

20. Fritillaria Extract Tablet 川 貝 精 片

Common Usages: For acute and chronic coughs accompanied by tightness in the chest, with or without symptoms of a cold. May also be used for bronchitis and mild asthma in children, and for the bronchial asthma associated with changes in climate.

Traditional Usages and Functions: Relieves cough, eliminates phlegm, and moistens Lungs.

English Transliteration: Fritillaria Extract Formula

Pinyin Mandarin Name: *Chuan Bei Jing Pian*

Forms Used: May be made into a tea or used in patent form.

Pinyin Name	Common English Name	Quantity in grams	Traditional Herb Function
Chuan bei mu	Fritillaria, bulb	4.0	Clears heat; transforms phlegm
Yuan zhi	Polygala, rt.	4.0	Expels phlegm from Lungs; clears orifices
Wu wei zi	Schisandra	3.5	Contains leakage of Lung Qi; stops cough

Pinyin Name	Common English Name	Quantity in grams	Traditional Herb Function
Jie geng	Platycodon, rt.	3.0	Circulates Lung Qi; moves other herbs upward
Chen pi	Citrus, pl. (aged)	3.0	Moves Qi; dries damp; transforms phlegm
Gan cao	Licorice, rx.	2.5	Moistens Lungs; stops coughing; harmonizes other herbs

NOTE: This formula is used most often to clear phlegm from the lungs, especially in combination with other herbal formulas such as Lonicera and Forsythia (*Yin Chiao Chieh Tu Pien*) if there are wind-heat symptoms such as sore throat, fever, and yellow phlegm; or Ma Huang Formula (*Ma Huang Tang*) if there are signs of wind cold such as tickle in the throat, achiness, chills, clear white phlegm, and no sweating.
Cautions in Use: None.

21. Gentiana Formula　　龍胆瀉肝丸

Common Usages: Used most often for acute and chronic Bladder conditions, such as cystitis, that may or may not be accompanied by vaginal discharge, burning urine, thirst, and itching in groin area. Other symptoms that may accompany a Bladder infection include headache, red eyes, bitter taste in mouth, fever blisters in mouth, dizziness, ringing and pain in the ears, pain in Stomach and/or rib area, difficulty urinating, and/or dark urine. Gentiana Formula has also been used to treat herpes of the mouth or genitals and hyperthyroidism.
Traditional Usages and Functions: Used for Liver and Gallbladder fire and dampness. Clears Liver and Gallbladder heat and moves dampness.
English Transliteration: Gentiana Formula
Pinyin Mandarin Name: *Long Dan Xie Gan Wan*
Forms Used: May be made into a tea or used in patent or granular forms.

Pinyin Name	Common English Name	Quantity in grams	Traditional Herb Function
Long dan cao	Gentian, rt.	1.0-3.0	Drains Liver and Gallbladder damp and fire
Ze xie	Alisma, rhz.	1.0-3.0	Removes dampness; drains Kidney fire

Pinyin Name	Common English Name	Quantity in grams	Traditional Herb Function
Mu tong	Akebia, stem	1.0	Promotes urination; drains heat
Che qian zi	Plantago, sd.	1.0	Promotes urination; clears heat
Tang gui	Angelica, rt.	4.0	Tonifies and invigorates Blood
Sheng di huang	Rehmannia, rt. (raw)	1.0-5.0	Cools upward Heart fire; nourishes yin
Zhi zi	Gardenia. fr.	1.0	Drains damp heat; cools Blood
Huang qin	Scutellaria, rx.	3.0	Clears heat; drains damp heat
Gan cao	Licorice, rx.	1.5	Tonifies Spleen; benefits Qi

Cautions in Use: Amount of raw herb in formula may have to be adjusted for level of dampness present. Do not use during pregnancy.

22. Ginseng and Astragalus Formula 補中益氣丸

Common Usages: For general fatigue with mild fever, sweating, and poor appetite. Also for headache with chills. Often used to strengthen digestive function and weakness asociated with the more chronic symptoms of Organ prolapse, hernia, hemorrhoids, varicose veins, and chronic diarrhea. Useful for low blood pressure.

Traditional Usages and Functions: Tonifies Qi, Spleen, and Stomach; raises Yang.

English Transliteration: Ginseng and Astragalus

Pinyin Mandarin Name: *Bu Zhong Yi Qi Wan*

Forms Used: May be made into a tea or used in patent or granular forms.

Pinyin Name	Common English Name	Quantity in grams	Traditional Herb Function
Ren shen	Ginseng, rx.	4.0	Tonifies Qi and Stomach; strengthens Spleen
Huang qi	Astragalus, rt.	4.0	Tonifies Spleen, Qi, and Blood; raises yang Qi
Gan cao	Licorice, rx.	1.5	Tonifies Spleen; benefits Qi

Pinyin Name	Common English Name	Quantity in grams	Traditional Herb Function
Bai zhu	Atractylodes, rhz.	4.0	Tonifies Spleen Qi; dries Dampness
Tang gui	Angelica, rt.	3.0	Tonifies and invigorates blood
Sheng jiang pi	Ginger, Fresh rhz.	1.0	Disperses cold; adjusts Nutritive Qi
Da zao	Ziziphi, fr.	2.0	Tonifies Spleen; benefits Stomach
Chen pi	Citrus, pl. (aged)	2.0	Move Qi; strengthens Stomach; stops vomiting
Chai hu	Bupleurum, rt.	2.0	Raises Spleen, Stomach, and yang Qi
Sheng ma	Cimicifuga, rt.	1.0	Raises yang Qi

Cautions in Use: Do not use when there is high blood pressure or bloating with hard abdomen.

23. Ginseng and Atractylodes Formula 参苓白术片

Common Usages: For chronic diarrhea; and for other gastrointestinal problems with poor appetite, fatigue and chills, indigestion, bloating, vomiting, and diarrhea. Also used for morning sickness; poor appetite in children; and the chronic intestinal problems associated with long-term illnesses such as chronic fatigue syndrome, fibromyalgia, HIV, and anemia.

Traditional Usages and Functions: Use for gastrointestinal weakness due to Spleen and Stomach Qi deficiency. Tonifies Stomach and Spleen Qi.

English Transliteration: Ginseng and Atractylodes

Pinyin Mandarin Name: *Shen Ling Bai Zhu Pian*

Forms Used: May be made into a tea or used in patent or granular forms.

Pinyin Name	Common English Name	Quantity in grams	Traditional Herb Function
Ren shen	Ginseng, rx.	3.0	Tonifies Qi and Stomach; strengthens Spleen
Bai zhu	Atractylodes, rhz.	3.0	Tonifies Spleen Qi; dries dampness

Pinyin Name	Common English Name	Quantity in grams	Traditional Herb Function
Fu ling	Poria (fungus)	3.0	Strengthens Spleen; moves dampness
Shan yao	Dioscoria, rx.	3.0	Tonifies Spleen Qi
Gan cao	Licorice, rx.	1.5	Tonifies Spleen; benefits Qi
Lian zi	Lotus Seed	4.0	Nourishes Kidneys; strengthens Spleen; stops diarrhea
Yi yi ren	Coix, sd.	5.0	Strengthens Spleen; moves dampness; stops diarrhea
Bai bian dou	Dolichos	4.0	Strengthens Spleen
Sha ren	Cardamom, sd.	2.0	Moves Qi; strengthens Stomach
Jie geng	Platycodon, rt.	2.0	Circulates Lung Qi; moves other herbs upward

Cautions in Use: Do not use at onset of cold or flu; may be used once recovery has begun.

24. Ginseng and Longan Formula 歸脾湯

Common Usages: For the gastrointestinal upsets, fatigue, anemia, palpitations, insomnia, sweating, absentmindedness, and/or neurosis associated with gastrointestinal weakness, major illness, or physical/emotional stress. Also used for heavy menstrual bleeding or spotting.

Traditional Usages and Functions: Often used for deficient Spleen Qi. Tonifies Qi and Blood; strengthens Spleen and spirit. May also be used to offset bloating associated with other tonifying formulas.

English Transliteration: Ginseng and Longan Formula

Pinyin Mandarin Name: *Gui Pi Tang*

Forms Used: May be made into a tea or used in patent or granular forms.

Pinyin Name	Common English Name	Quantity in grams	Traditional Herb Function
Ren shen	Ginseng, rx.	2.0-3.0	Tonifies Qi and Stomach; strengthens Spleen
Fu ling	Poria (fungus)	3.0	Strengthens Spleen; moves dampness

Pinyin Name	Common English Name	Quantity in grams	Traditional Herb Function
Bai zhu	Atractylodes, rhz.	3.0	Tonifies Spleen Qi; dries Dampness
Gan cao	Licorice, rx.	1.0	Tonifies Spleen; benefits Qi
Tang gui	Angelica, rt.	2.0	Tonifies and invigorates Blood
Da zao	Ziziphi, fr.	1.0	Tonifies Spleen; benefits Stomach
Suan zao ren	Ziziphi, sd.	3.0	Nourishes Heart and Liver; calms spirit
Huang qi	Astragalus, rt.	2.0	Tonifies Spleen, Qi, and Blood; raises yang Qi
Long yan rou	Longan, fr.	3.0	Tonifies Heart and Spleen; calms spirit
Yuan zhi	Polygala, rt.	1.0	Calms spirit; expels phlegm
Mu xiang	Saussurea, rt.	1.0	Moves and regulates Qi; strengthens Spleen
Sheng jiang pi	Ginger, fresh rhz.	1.0	Disperses cold; adjusts Nutritive Qi

Cautions in Use: Do not use at onset of cold or flu; may be used once recovery has begun.

25. Ginseng and Tang Gui Ten Formula 十 全 大 補 丸

Common Usages: Used for poor or no appetite with gastrointestinal weakness, muscle spasms and/or pain, chills, rough skin, fatigue, weak back and/or legs, shortness of breath, palpitations, and anxiety. Often used after surgery or major illness to strengthen general health and enhance recovery.

Traditional Usages and Functions: Tonifies Qi and Blood; warms the body.

English Transliteration: Ginseng Tang Gui Ten Formula

Pinyin Mandarin Name: *Shi Quan Da Bu Wan*

Forms Used: May be made into a tea or used in patent or granular forms.

Pinyin Name	Common English Name	Quantity in grams	Traditional Herb Function
Ren shen	Ginseng, rx.	3.0	Tonifies Qi and Stomach; strengthens Spleen
Haung qi	Astragalus, rt.	3.0	Tonifies Spleen, Qi, and Blood; raises yang Qi
Bai shao	Peony Alba, rx.	3.0	Pacifies Liver; Tonifies Blood; preserves yin
Bai zhu	Atractylodes, rhz.	3.0	Tonifies Spleen Qi; dries dampness
Fu ling	Poria (fungus)	3.0	Strengthens Spleen; moves dampness
Shu di huang	Rehmannia (steamed)	4.0	Tonifies Liver and Kidneys; nourishes yin
Tang gui	Angelica, rt.	4.0	Tonifies and invigorates Blood
Rou gui	Cinnamon, rx.	1.5	Warms Kidney yang
Chuan xiang	Ligusticum, rhz.	2.0	Invigorates Blood; moves Qi
Gan cao	Licorice, rx.	1.0	Tonifies Spleen; benefits Qi

Cautions in Use: Do not use with high blood pressure or during pregnancy. Avoid in cases where person always feels hot. Do not use at onset of colds or the flu, but may be used once recovery has begun.

26. Ginseng and Zizyphus Formula 天王補心丹

Common Usages: For insomnia, heart palpitations, disturbed sleep with vivid dreams, anxiety, restlessness, and forgetfulness. Also used for hyperactive thyroid and for dry stools.

Traditional Usages and Functions: Nourishes Yin and Blood; calms Heart and Shen (spirit).

English Transliteration: Ginseng and Zizyphus

Pinyin Mandarin Name: *Tian Wang Bu Xin Dan*

Forms Used: May be made into a tea or used in patent or granular forms.

Pinyin Name	Common English Name	Quantity in grams	Traditional Herb Function
Sheng di huang	Rehmannia, rt. (raw)	6.0	Cools upward Heart fire; nourishes yin

Pinyin Name	Common English Name	Quantity in grams	Traditional Herb Function
Ren shen	Ginseng, rx.	1.0	Tonifies Qi and Stomach; strengthens Spleen
Xuan shen	Scrophularia, rx.	2.0	Nourishes yin; cools Blood
Wu wei zi	Schisandra, fr.	2.0	Contains leakage of Lung Qi; stops cough
Tian men dong	Asparagus, rx.	2.0	Moistens Lungs; nourishes Kidneys; cools heat
Tang gui	Angelica, rt.	2.0	Tonifies and invigorates Blood
Mai men dong	Ophiopogon, rt.	2.0	Nourishes yin; moistens Lungs; stop cough
Bai zi ren	Biota, sd.	2.0	Nourishes Heart; calms spirit
Suan zao ren	Zizyphi, sd.	2.0	Nourishes Heart and Liver; calms spirit
Yuan zhi	Polygala, rt.	1.0	Calms spirit; expels phlegm
Dan shen	Salvia, rt.	1.0	Invigorates Blood; clears heat
Jie geng	Platycodon, rt.	1.0	Circulates Lung Qi; moves other herbs upward

Cautions in Use: Make sure that dampness is under control before using this formula for an extended period of time, and watch for signs that dampness may be becoming a problem. Avoid greasy foods and excessive dairy products when using this formula. Do not use at onset of colds or the flu, but may be used once recovery has begun.

27. Hoelen and Polyporus Formula 治濁固本丸

Common Usages: For chronic urethritis, cystitis, and prostatitis, or any prostate imbalance. Also used for chronic leakage of seminal fluid. Reduces inflammation and promotes urination.

Traditional Usages and Functions: For heat and dampness in the Bladder and prostate with turbid or white urine. Clears heat; dispels dampness; clears turbidity; reduces inflammation; promotes urination.

English Transliteration: Hoelen and Polyporus
Pinyin Mandarin Name: *Zhi Zhuo Gu Ben Wan*
Forms Used: May be made into a tea or used in granular form.

Pinyin Name	Common English Name	Quantity in grams	Traditional Herb Function
Huang lian	Coptis, rhz.	2.0	Clears heat; drains dampness
Fu ling	Poria/Hoelen (fungus)	1.0	Promotes urination; leaches dampness
Zhu ling	Grifola (fungus)	2.0	Promotes urination; leaches dampness
Sha ren	Cardamom, sd.	1.0	Moves Qi; strengthens Stomach
Ban xia	Pinellia, rhz.	1.0	Dries damp; transforms phlegm; calms Stomach
Lian xu	Nelumbinus, stamen	2.0	Stabilizes Kidneys; retains Essence
Yi zhi ren	Cardamom (black), sd.	1.0	Warms Kidneys; retains Essence
Gan cao	Licorice, rx.	3.0	Tonifies Spleen; benefits Qi, soothes spasm
Huang bai	Phellodendron, bk.	1.0	Drains damp heat; quells Kidney fire

Cautions in Use: Before using this formula, it is important to rule out acute inflammations and/or malignancies. Do not use during pregnancy.

28. Hoelin Five Formula   五苓散

Common Usages: Used for surface flu symptoms such as headache, fever, thirst (but vomiting after drinking), combined with inability to urinate, swelling of legs and lower body, diarrhea, vertigo, palpitations, and overall dehydration exacerbated by vomiting. May also be used for motion sickness, toxemia during pregnancy, cardiac edema, chronic headache, and some cases of trigeminal neuralgia.
Traditional Usages and Functions: Clears heat and dampness, promotes urination, and warms Yang.
English Transliteration: Hoelin Five Formula
Pinyin Mandarin Name: *Wu Lin San*
Forms Used: May be made into a tea or used in granular form.

Pinyin Name	Common English Name	Quantity in grams	Traditional Herb Function
Ze xie	Alismatis, rhz.	6.0	Removes dampness; drains Kidney fire
Zhu ling	Grifola (fungus)	4.5	Promotes urination; leaches out dampness
Fu ling	Poria/Hoelen (fungus)	3.0	Strengthens Spleen; promotes urination
Bai zhu	Atractylodes, rhz.	1.0	Tonifies Spleen Qi; resolves dampness
Gui zhi	Cinnamon, twig	4.0	Warms channels; warms yang; moves damp

Cautions in Use: None.

29. Ilex and Evodia Formula　　感冒靈

Common Usages: For colds, flus, and other viruses with symptoms of chills, high fever, swollen lymph glands, sore throat, and stiffness of the upper back and neck. Most effective when used at the first signs of cold and/or flu symptoms.

Traditional Usages and Functions: Used for both wind-cold and wind-heat syndromes. Dispels wind, sedates heat.

English Transliteration: Common Cold Effective Remedy

Pinyin Mandarin Name: *Ganmaoling*

Forms Used: May be made into a tea or used in patent form.

Pinyin Name	Common English Name	Quantity in grams	Traditional Herb Function
Kang mei ken	Ilex Asperella	3.5	Dispels heat; removes toxins
San ya ku	Evodia, fr.	2.5	Remove toxins; expels wind and dampness
Jin yin hua	Lonicera, fl.	0.5	Clears heat; detoxifies fire poison
Ban lan gen	Isatidis, rt.	1.5	Quells heat; benefits throat
Huang jing zi	Viticus Negundinis, fr.	1.5	Dispels wind; resolves phlegm
Ye ju hua	Chrysanthemum, wild	1.5	Quells fire; detoxifies fire poison
Bo he nao	Menthol, crystal	0.0001	Opens orifices

Cautions in Use: Do not use during pregnancy.

30. Leonuris and Achyranthes Formula 降壓丸

Common Usages: For acute or chronic high blood pressure (hypertension), particularly when associated with central-nervous-system disorders such as severe headache, vertigo, facial paralysis, numbness, and/or speech difficulties. Other associated symptoms may include stiff neck, red face, diminished vision, and/or abnormal sensations in face or limbs.

Traditional Usages and Functions: Clears heat, calms internal wind, and promotes circulation.

English Transliteration: Leonuris and Achyranthes Formula (Hypertension Pills)

Pinyin Mandarin Name: *Jiang Ya Wan*

Forms Used: May be made into a tea or used in patent form.

Pinyin Name	Common English Name	Quantity in grams	Traditional Herb Function
Yi mu cao	Leonuris, sd., hb.	5.0	Invigorates Blood; promotes urination
Huang lian	Coptis, rhz.	1.0	Clears heat; clears Heart fire
Ling yang jiao	Antelope horn	1.0	Pacifies Liver; extinguishes wind
Gou teng	Uncaria	2.5	Extinguishes wind; quells heat; pacifies Liver; lowers blood pressure
Hu po	Amber, resin	1.0	Promotes urination; invigorates Blood; calms spirit
Tang gui	Angelica, rt.	2.5	Tonifies and invigorates Blood
Chen xiang	Aquilaria, wood	2.0	Moves stagnant Qi
Chuan xiang	Ligusticum, rhz.	2.0	Invigorates Blood; moves Qi
Tian ma	Gastrodia, rhz.	1.5	Pacifies Liver; extinguishes wind
Da huang	Rhubarb, rhz.	1.5	Drains damp heat; drains excess heat from Blood
Sheng di huang	Rehmannia, rt. (raw)	3.0	Cools upward Heart fire; nourishes yin
E jiao	Gelatin, skin	3.0	Nourishes Blood and yin

Pinyin Name	Common English Name	Quantity in grams	Traditional Herb Function
Xia ku cao	Prunella, spike	2.0	Clears Liver; disperses Liver fire; lowers blood pressure
Mu dan pi	Moutan, cx. rx.	2.0	Drains Liver fire; cools Blood; lowers blood pressure
Niu xi	Achyranthes, rt.	4.5	Invigorates Blood; dispels clots

NOTE: *Jiang Ya Wan* is a patent medicine made in Beijing, China. A similar formulation (*Chiang Ya Pien*) is made in Hopei province and may be easier to obtain. It has similar functions to *Jiang Ya Wan* and may be used for the same basic imbalances.

Cautions in Use: Do not use during pregnancy. This formula may cause loose stools. As in all cases involving serious imbalances, care should be taken to continue taking conventional medication and to slowly withdraw from conventional medicines only under the careful supervision of your practitioner.

31. Lonicera and Forsythia Formula   銀翹解毒片

Common Usages: For early symptoms of seasonal cold and flu viruses, including swollen lymph nodes, body and joint aches, fever, chills, headache, sore throat, stiff neck, sparse perspiration, and associated rashes and hives. Also used for early symptoms of measles, mumps, and tonsilitis.

Traditional Usages and Functions: Used to relieve and clear toxic wind-heat symptoms. Promotes sweating.

English Transliteration: Lonicera and Forsythia Formula

Pinyin Mandarin Name: *Yin Chiao Chieh Tu Pien*

Forms Used: May be made into a tea or used in patent or granular forms.

Pinyin Name	Common English Name	Quantity in grams	Traditional Herb Function
Jin yin hua	Lonicera, fl.	3.0	Clears surface heat; detoxifies fire poison
Lian qiao	Forsythia, fr.	3.0	Expels externally contracted wind heat
Jie geng	Platycodon, rt.	2.0	Circulates Lung Qi; benefits throat

Pinyin Name	Common English Name	Quantity in grams	Traditional Herb Function
Bo he	Peppermint, leaf	2.0	Disperses wind heat; benefits throat
Dan zhu ye	Bamboo, leaf	1.5	Releases exterior; disperses wind heat
Gan cao	Licorice, rx.	1.5	Moistens Lungs; stops coughing; harmonizes other herbs
Jing jie	Schizonepeta, hb.	1.0	Releases exterior; expels wind
Dan dou chi	Soja, sd. (prepared)	1.5	Releases exterior; alleviates irritability
Niu bang zi	Burdock, fr.	1.5	Disperses wind heat; benefits throat

Cautions in Use: *Yin Chiao* is also available in a commercially prepared, sugarcoated version that contains caffeine, paracetamolum, and chlorpheniraminum. You may wish to avoid this formulation.

32. Ma Huang Formula   麻黃湯

Common Usages: For seasonal viruses with accompanying body ache, headache, chest distension, cough with tickle in the throat, runny nose, and chills; for acute and chronic bronchitis and asthmas; and for the symptoms of seasonal allergies such as hay fever that have runny nose with clear phlegm.

Traditional Usages and Functions: Used for wind-cold surface symptoms. Relieves exterior heat; promotes sweating; promotes circulation of Lung Qi; relieves asthma.

English Transliteration: Ma Huang Formula

Pinyin Mandarin Name: *Ma Huang Tang*

Forms Used: May be made into a tea or used in granular forms.

Pinyin Name	Common English Name	Quantity in grams	Traditional Herb Function
Ma huang	Ephedra, hb.	5.0	Releases exterior; disperses cold; circulates Lung Qi
Gui zhi	Cinnamon, twig	4.0	Warms channels; disperses cold and pain

Pinyin Name	Common English Name	Quantity in grams	Traditional Herb Function
Xing ren	Apricot, sd.	5.0	Relieves cough; stops wheezing
Gan cao	Licorice, rx.	1.5	Moistens Lungs; stops coughing; harmonizes other herbs

Cautions in Use: Ma Huang has a mildly stimulative effect. To prevent sleep difficulties, avoid use in the evenings. Do not use when person has palpitation or has a nervous personality. Do not use during pregnacy.

33. Major Four Herbs Formula　四君子湯

Common Usage: A general strengthening tonic for individuals who have overworked, underslept, and eaten poorly. Associated symptoms often include poor appetite, loose stools, poor muscle tone, pale complexion, and low/soft voice. An individual presenting with the latter symptoms may be at risk for irritable bowel syndrome, chronic gastritis, peptic ulcers, and/or diabetes.

Traditional Usages and Functions: Tonifies Qi and strengthens Spleen.

English Transliteration: Major Four Herbs Formula

Pinyin Mandarin Name: *Si Jun Zi Tang*

Forms Used: May be made into a tea or used in patent or granular forms.

Pinyin Name	Common English Name	Quantity in grams	Traditional Herb Function
Ren shen	Ginseng, rx.	4.0	Tonifies Original Qi; strengthens Stomach and Spleen; benefits Heart Qi
Bai zhu	Atractylodes, rhz.	4.0	Tonifies Spleen Qi; dries dampness
Fu ling	Poria (fungus)	4.0	Strengthens Spleen; harmonizes Middle Burner
Zhi gan cao	Licorice, honey-baked	1.5	Tonifies Spleen; benefits Qi

Cautions in Use: Do not use with high fever. Do not use with signs of deficient heat or strong Yin deficiency. Overuse of this formula may result in dry mouth, thirst, and irritability.

34. Major Six Herbs Formula 六君子湯

Common Usages: For symptoms of poor digestion accompanied by poor appetite, loose stools, acid reflux, nausea, and vomiting. Other associated symptoms may include fatigue, anemia, cold hands and feet, and a sensation of fullness beneath the heart.

Traditional Usages and Functions: For symptoms of Spleen dampness. Tonifies Qi, strengthens Spleen, and dispels moisture.

English Transliteration: Major Six Herbs Formula

Pinyin Mandarin Name: *Liu Jun Zi Tang*

Forms Used: May be made into a tea or used in patent or granular forms.

Pinyin Name	Common English Name	Quantity in grams	Traditional Herb Function
Ren shen	Ginseng, rx.	4.0	Tonifies Original Qi; strengthens Stomach and Spleen; benefits Heart Qi
Bai Zhu	Atractylodes, rhz.	4.0	Tonifies Spleen Qi; dries dampness
Fu ling	Poria (fungus)	4.0	Strengthens Spleen; harmonizes Middle Burner
Zhi gan cao	Licorice, honey-baked	1.0	Tonifies Spleen; benefits Qi
Chen pi	Citrus, pl. (aged)	2.0	Moves Qi; strengthens Stomach; stops vomiting
Ban xia	Pinellia, rhz.	4.0	Dries damp; transforms phlegm; calms Stomach
Sheng jiang	Ginger, fresh rhz.	2.0	Disperses cold; adjusts Nutritive Qi
Da zao	Ziziphi, fr.	2.0	Tonifies Spleen; benefits Stomach

NOTE: Codonopsis (*dang shen*) is often substituted for ginseng in this formula and in patent formulas. Ginger (*sheng jiang*) and ziziphus jujube (*da zao*) are also often omitted.

Cautions in Use: None.

35. Minor Bupleurum Formula 小柴胡湯

Common Usages: This formula is used for stress-related abdominal problems, including alternating chills and fever with a sensation of heaviness and pain below the ribs, often accompanied by a bitter or sour taste in mouth with dry throat and dizziness, nausea and vomiting, poor appetite, and heartburn; also used for gallstones, intercostal neuralgia, flu, jaundice, and the generalized weakness that follows such conditions.

Traditional Usages and Functions: Soothes Liver; cleanses Gallbladder; treats deep, but not-yet-seated, invasion of disease.

English Transliteration: Minor Bupleurum Formula

Pinyin Mandarin Name: *Xiao Chai Hu Tang*

Forms Used: May be made into a tea or used in granular form.

Pinyin Name	Common English Name	Quantity in grams	Traditional Herb Function
Chai hu	Bupleurum, rt.	7.0	Resolves lesser yang heat patterns; relaxes Liver Qi
Huang qin	Scutellaria, rx.	3.0	Clears heat; drains damp heat
Ban xia	Pinellia, rhz.	5.0	Dries damp; transforms phlegm; calms Stomach
Sheng jiang	Ginger, fresh rhz.	4.0	Disperses cold; adjusts Nutritive Qi
Ren shen	Ginseng, rx.	3.0	Tonifies Qi and Stomach; strengthens Spleen
Da zao	Ziziphi, fr.	3.0	Tonifies Spleen; benefits Stomach; calms Spirit
Gan cao	Licorice, rx.	2.0	Tonifies Qi; harmonizes herbs

Cautions in Use: Use cautiously where there is hypertension or vomiting of blood due to Yin deficiency. This formula should not be taken long term.

36. Panax Ginseng Capsules 長白山人參丸

Common Usages: Used as a tonic to strengthen immune function, digestion, and energy levels; helps the body to adapt to adverse circumstances and increases the body's resistance.

Traditional Usages and Functions: Tonifies Qi. When used in other formulas, it strengthens the Qi-tonifying effects of other herbs.
English Transliteration: Ginseng Capsules
Pinyin Mandarin Name: *Renshen Wan*
Forms Used: May be used as a tea or in patent form.

Pinyin Name	Common English Name	Quantity in grams	Traditional Herb Function
Ren shen	Ginseng, rx.	1.0	Tonifies Original Qi; strengthens Stomach and Spleen; benefits Heart Qi

Cautions in Use: Do not use during pregnancy. Do not use during the beginning stages of a cold or respiratory disorder. There is a possibility that this herb will enhance the effect of the disorder. As a result, it is best taken when one is "over the hump" and on the road to recovery, at which time it will speed recovery.

37. Peony and Licorice Formula   芍药甘草湯

Common Usages: Soothe the spasms associated with many muscular disorders, as well as spasms associated with fluid loss due to sweating, diarrhea, and/or blood loss. Also has been used to treat intercostal neuralgia, sciatica, trigeminal neuralgia, intestinal colic, children's colic, menstrual spasms, and smooth muscle spasms of the stomach, intestines, Gallbladder, and ureter.
Traditional Usages and Functions: To relieve Blood deficiency–related muscle spasms and pain.
English Transliteration: Peony and Licorice Formula
Pinyin Mandarin Name: *Shao Yao Gan Cao Tang*
Forms Used: May be made into a tea or used in granular form.

Pinyin Name	Common English Name	Quantity in grams	Traditional Herb Function
Bai shao	Peony Alba, rx.	6.0	Pacifies Liver; alleviates pain
Gan cao	Licorice, rx.	6.0	Tonifies Spleen; benefits Qi; soothes spasms

Cautions in Use: None.

38. Polygonum Tablet 首烏片

Common Usages: For general lack of vitality, with headaches, dizziness, eye pain, low back pain, and/or painful joints. Also used for menstrual difficulties. Most frequently—and famously—prescribed for premature and early stage of greying hair.

Traditional Usages and Functions: Used for chronic deficiences of Liver Blood and Liver Fire. Nourishes Liver Blood and tonifies Kidney Qi and Jing (essence). *He shou wu pian* is one of the few Chinese herbs used alone.For insomnia, heart palpitations.

English Transliteration: Polygonum Tablet

Pinyin Mandarin Name: *He Shou Wu Pian*

Forms Used: May be made into a tea or used in patent or granular forms.

Pinyin Name	Common English Name	Quantity in grams	Traditional Herb Function
He shou wu	Polygonum Multiflorum, hb.	3.0-10.0	Tonifies Liver and Kidneys; nourishes Blood

Cautions in Use: None.

39. Prunella and Scutellaria Formula 降壓平片

Common Usages: For lowering blood pressure and reducing cholesterol. Especially effective if treatment is started early, before hardening of plaque. Also has been used to treat dizziness, ringing in the ears, headache, agitation, and stress-related hypertension.

Traditional Usages and Functions: For symptoms of Liver fire and internal wind. Sedates Liver fire and calms internal Liver wind.

English Transliteration: Hypertension Repressing Tablets

Pinyin Mandarin Name: *Jiang Ya Ping Pian*

Forms Used: May be made into a tea or used in patent form.

Pinyin Name	Common English Name	Quantity in grams	Traditional Herb Function
Xia ku cao	Prunella, spike	5.0	Clears Liver; disperses Liver fire; lowers blood pressure
Huang qin	Scutellaria, rx.	5.0	Clears heat; disperses fire

Pinyin Name	Common English Name	Quantity in grams	Traditional Herb Function
Di long	Lumbricus	4.0	Clears Liver heat; calms wind
Ju hua	Chrysanthemum, fl.	2.0	Cools Liver heat; extinguishes wind
Huai hua mi	Sophora, imm. fl.	2.0	Cools Liver heat; cools Blood; lowers blood pressure

NOTE: This formula can and should regularly be taken for several months or even years. It is often combined with the Leonuris and Achyranthes Formula (*Jiang Ya Wan*) in more advanced or chronic cases of hypertension, or where there is a history of strokes or mini-strokes.

Cautions in Use: As in all cases involving serious imbalances, care should be taken to continue taking conventional medication, and to slowly withdraw from conventional medicine only under the careful supervision of your practitioners. Do not use during pregnancy.

40. Pseudoginseng and Dragon Blood Formula   筋骨跌傷丸

Common Usages: For traumatic injuries including fracture, sprains, strains, and wounds accompanied by pain and swelling; stops internal bleeding; helps bones and tendons knit more rapidly; alleviates pain.

Traditional Usages and Functions: Reduces swelling; stops bleeding; moves Blood stagnation; promotes healing.

English Transliteration: Pseudoginseng and Dragon Blood Formula

Pinyin Mandarin Name: *Chin Koo Tieh Shang Wan*

Forms Used: May be made into a tea or used in patent form.

Pinyin Name	Common English Name	Quantity in grams	Traditional Herb Function
Tian qi	Pseudoginseng, rt.	6.0	Reduces swelling; alleviates pain; moves Blood stagnation
Xue jie	Dragon Blood	5.0	Moves congealed Blood; alleviates pain; stops bleeding
Tang gui	Angelica, rt.	4.0	Tonifies and invigorates Blood

Pinyin Name	Common English Name	Quantity in grams	Traditional Herb Function
Ru xiang	Frankincense, gum	3.0	Invigorates Blood; alleviates pain; promotes healing
Mo yao	Myrrh, gum	2.5	Moves congealed Blood; alleviates pain; promotes healing
Hong hua	Carthamus, fl.	2.5	Dispels congealed Blood; alleviates pain

Cautions in Use: Do not use during pregnancy.

41. Pueraria Combination　　葛根湯

Common Usages: For colds with chills—with or without fever—accompanied by stiffness in neck and upper back, congestion, muscle spasms, and headache.

Traditional Usages and Functions: Relieves external symptoms and muscle aches; harmonizes Nutritive and Protective Qi.

English Transliteration: Pueraria Formula

Pinyin Mandarin Name: *Ge Gen Tang*

Forms Used: May be used as a tea or in patent or granular forms.

Pinyin Name	Common English Name	Quantity in grams	Traditional Herb Function
Ge gen	Pueraria, rt.	8.0	Releases muscles; clears heat
Bai shao	Peony Alba, rx.	3.0	Adjusts Nutritive and Protective Qi levels
Gui zhi	Cinnamon, twig	3.0	Warms channels; disperses cold
Ma huang	Ephedra, hb.	4.0	Releases exterior; disperses cold; circulates Lung Qi
Sheng jiang	Ginger, fresh rhz.	1.0	Disperses cold; adjusts Nutritive Qi
Da zao	Ziziphi, fr.	4.0	Tonifies Spleen; benefits Stomach
Gan cao	Licorice, rx.	2.0	Moistens Lungs; stops coughing; harmonizes other herbs

Cautions in Use: Do not use during pregnancy.

42. Qiang-Huo and Turmeric Formula 蠲痹湯

Common Usages: Used chiefly for joint pain and stiffness, especially shoulder-joint pain and stiffness, and the wrist pain associated with carpal tunnel syndrome. Also used for neck and upper-back spasms with difficulty in movement, and for pain in limbs and waist.

Traditional Usages and Functions: Tonifies Qi; activates Blood; dispels wind; removes dampness.

English Transliteration: Qiang-Huo and Turmeric Formula
Pinyin Mandarin Name: *Jian Pi Tang*
Forms Used: May be made into a tea or used in granular form.

Pinyin Name	Common English Name	Quantity in grams	Traditional Herb Function
Qiang-huo	Angelica sylvestris, rt. stalk	4.5	Releases exterior; disperses cold and damp; penetrates obstruction; alleviates pain
Jiang huang	Curcuma, rhz.	4.5	Moves Qi; alleviates pain
Tang gui	Angelica, rt.	4.5	Tonifies and invigorates Blood
Chi shao	Peony Rubra, rx.	4.5	Invigorates Blood; dispels congealed Blood
Huang qi	Astragalus, rt.	4.5	Tonifies Spleen; benefits Qi
Fang feng	Siler, rt.	4.5	Expels wind dampness; alleviates pain
Gan cao	Licorice, rx.	1.5	Tonifies Qi; benefits Spleen; soothes spasms
Sheng jiang	Ginger, fresh rhz.	1.0	Disperses cold; adjusts Nutritive Qi
Da zao	Ziziphi, fr.	1.0	Tonifies Spleen; benefits Stomach

Cautions in Use: Do not use during pregnancy.

43. Rehmannia and Dogwood Fruit Formula 明目地黃丸

Common Usages: For symptoms of night blindness; photophobia; dryness of eyes; tears on exposure to wind; glaucoma; cataracts; blurred vision; and chronic redness and weakness of eyes.

Traditional Usages and Functions: Used for deficiencies of Liver and Kidney Yin. Nourishes Liver and Kidney to improve eyesight.
English Transliteration: Rehmannia and Dogwood Fruit Combination
Pinyin Mandarin Name: *Ming Mu Di Huang Wan*
Forms Used: May be made into a tea or used in patent or granular form.

Pinyin Name	Common English Name	Quantity in grams	Traditional Herb Function
Shu di huang	Rehmannia (steamed)	4.0	Tonifies Liver and Kidneys; nourishes Yin
Ze xie	Alisma, rhz.	3.0	Purges fire; helps Rehmannia
Sahn zhu yu	Cornus, fr.	3.0-4.5	Nourishes Liver; astringes essence
Mu dan pi	Moutan, cx. rx.	3.0	Drains Liver fire; cools Blood
Shan yao	Dioscoria, rx.	3.0-4.5	Tonifies Spleen Qi
Fu ling	Poria (fungus)	3.0	Strengthens Spleen; moves dampness
Gou qi zi	Lycium, fr.	3.0-4.5	Nourishes Kidney and Liver yin; brightens eyes
Tang gui	Angelica, rt.	4.0	Tonifies and invigorates Blood
Ci ji li	Tribulus, fr.	3.0	Brightens eyes; smoothes Qi
Ju hua	Chrysanthemum, fl.	2.0	Cools Liver heat; brightens eyes
Bai shao	Peony Alba, rx.	3.0	Pacifies Liver; tonifies Blood; preserves Yin
Shi jue ming	Haliotidis, shell	5.0	Pacifies Liver Yang

Cautions in Use: Not useful with acute eye problems. Be careful if there is low blood pressure.

44. Rehmannia and Magnetitum Formula 耳鳴左慈丸

Common Usages: For ringing in the ears and other hearing difficulties, sometimes accompanied by vertigo, blurred vision, and other sensory disturbances.

Traditional Usages and Functions: For Kidney yin disturbances specifically associated with ringing in the ears. Nourishes yin and reduces Liver Yang.

English Transliteration: Rehmannia and Magnetitum Formula

Pinyin Mandarin Name: *Er Ming Zuo Ci Wan*

Forms Used: May be made into a tea or used in patent form.

Pinyin Name	Common English Name	Quantity in grams	Traditional Herb Function
Shu di huang	Rehmannia (steamed)	4.0	Tonifies Liver and Kidneys; nourishes yin
Ze xie	Alismatis, rhz.	1.5	Removes dampness; drains Kidney fire
Shan zhu yu	Cornus, fr.	2.0	Nourishes Liver; astringes Essence
Mu dan pi	Moutan, cx. rx.	1.5	Drains Liver fire; cools Blood
Shan yao	Dioscoria, rx.	2.0	Tonifies Spleen Qi
Fu ling	Poria (fungus)	1.5	Strengthens Spleen; moves dampness
Ci shi	Magnetititum	0.5	Sedates Heart; calms Spirit
Chai hu	Bupleurum, rt.	0.5	Relaxes constrained Liver Qi

Cautions in Use: Do not use during pregnancy.

45. Rehmannia Eight   八 味 地 黄 丸

Common Usages: For cold feet, knees, and hands; fatigue; inability to get or stay warm; frequent urination or poor urination; lower-back pain; swelling of the legs.

Traditional Usages and Functions: Rehmannia Eight is used for Kidney yang disturbances and deficiencies and for chronic, deep-seated deficiencies, also known as "life-gate deficiencies." It warms and supplements Kidney yang, and nourishes Yin and Jing (essence).

English Transliteration: Rehmannia Eight

Pinyin Mandarin Name: *Ba Wei Di Huang Wan*

Forms Used: May be made into a tea or used in patent or granular form.

Pinyin Name	Common English Name	Quantity in grams	Traditional Herb Function
Shu di huang	Rehmannia (steamed)	4.0	Tonifies Liver and Kidneys; nourishes yin
Ze xie	Alisma, rhz.	3.0	Purges fire; help Rehmannia
Sahn zhu yu	Cornus, fr.	3.0-4.5	Nourishes Liver; astringes essence
Mu dan pi	Moutan, cx. rx.	3.0	Drains Liver fire; cools Blood
Shan yao	Dioscoria, rx.	3.0-4.5	Tonifies Spleen Qi
Fu ling	Poria (fungus)	3.0	Strengthens Spleen; moves dampness
Rou gui	Cinnamon, rx.	1.0	Warms Kidney yang
Fu zi	Aconite (prepared)	1.0	Warms Kidney yang

Cautions in Use: Not for use by people who are always hot, or if there is high blood pressure.

46. Rehmannia Six　六味地黄丸

Common Usages: Ringing in the ears; poor hearing; night sweats; light-headedness; sore and weak lower back and knees; hot palms and soles; chronic sore throat; nocturnal emissions; and impotence.

Traditional Usages and Functions: Nourishes Kidney- and Liver-yin. Rehmannia Six is most often used for symptoms of Kidney- and Liver-yin deficiency and is useful in balancing yin deficiency and false Liver fire symptoms due to overuse of concentrated medications or vitamins.

English Transliteration: Rehmannia Six

Pinyin Mandarin Name: *Liu Wei Di Huang Wan*

Forms Used: May be made into a tea or used in patent or granular form.

Pinyin Name	Common English Name	Quantity in grams	Traditional Herb Function
Shu di huang	Rehmannia (steamed)	4.0	Tonifies Liver and Kidneys; nourishes yin
Ze xie	Alisma, rhz.	1.0-3.0	Removes dampness; drains Kidney fire
Sahn zhu yu	Cornus, fr.	3.0-4.5	Nourishes Liver; astringes Essence

Pinyin Name	Common English Name	Quantity in grams	Traditional Herb Function
Mu dan pi	Moutan, cx. rx.	3.0	Drains Liver fire; cools Blood
Shan yao	Dioscoria, rx.	3.0-4.5	Tonifies Spleen Qi
Fu ling	Poria (fungus)	3.0	Strengthens Spleen; moves dampness

Cautions in Use: Be careful when using Rehmannia Six if there is a white, greasy, coated tongue or other signs of dampness, digestive disturbances, or diarrhea due to a Spleen deficiency. Yin deficiency is one of the most prevalent imbalances in today's world, given the abundance of concentrated medications and foods, combined with hectic lifestyles. It is important to make sure that dampness is under control before using this formula for any extended period of time, and to watch for signs that it may be becoming a problem. To help with this, avoid greasy foods and excessive dairy products when using this formula.

47. Rhubarb and Scutellaria Formula   利胆片

Common Usages: For use in acute and chronic conditions of gallstone inflammation where small or sandy gallstones are present. May also be used for inflammation after gallstones are passed.

Traditional Usages and Functions: Resolves damp and toxic heat in the Liver and Gallbladder.

English Transliteration: Rhubarb and Scutellaria

Pinyin Mandarin Name: *Li Dan Pian*

Forms Used: May be made into a tea or used in patent or granular forms.

Pinyin Name	Common English Name	Quantity in grams	Traditional Herb Function
Huang qin	Scutellaria, rx.	3.0	Clears heat; drains damp heat
Mu xiang	Saussurea, rt.	1.5	Moves and regulates Qi; strengthens Spleen
Jin qian cao	Lysimachia (Desmodium)	1.0	Expels stones; clears Liver heat
Jin yin hua	Lonicera, fl.	1.0	Clears heat; detoxifies fire poison

Pinyin Name	Common English Name	Quantity in grams	Traditional Herb Function
Yin chen hao	Artemisia capillaris, hb.	1.0	Clears damp heat from Liver and Gallbladder; relieves jaundice
Chai hu	Bupleurum, rt.	2.0	Raises Spleen and Stomach yang Qi
Da huang	Rhubarb, Rhz.	0.5	Drains damp heat; detoxifies fire poison

Cautions in Use: When gallstones are present, it is best to have conventional screening to determine size and placement of stones. If large stones are lodged in duct, surgery may be necessary. Do not use during pregnancy.

48. Stephania and Astragalus Formula 防己黄耆湯

Common Usages: For poor circulation and edema in lower limbs accompanied by pale skin, soft muscles, water retention, profuse sweating with chills, lack of urination, and/or a sensation of heaviness. Arthritis, particularly of the knees, and/or irregular menstruation may also be present. Frequently prescribed for overweight people with latter conditions who have had trouble losing weight on conventional diets.

Traditional Usages and Functions: Tonifies Qi, strengthens Spleen, and reduces edema.

English Transliteration: Stephania and Astragalus

Pinyin Mandarin Name: *Fang Ji Huang Qi Tang*

Forms Used: May be made into a tea or used in granular form.

Pinyin Name	Common English Name	Quantity in grams	Traditional Herb Function
Han fang ji	Stephania, rt.	5.0	Expels wind dampness; promotes urination; reduces edema
Bai zhu	Atractylodes, rhz.	3.0	Tonifies Spleen Qi; resolves dampness
Huang qi	Astragalus, rt.	5.0	Tonifies Qi; strengthens surface; promotes urination
Gan cao	Licorice, rx.	1.5	Tonifies Qi; harmonizes other herbs

Pinyin Name	Common English Name	Quantity in grams	Traditional Herb Function
Da zao	Ziziphus, fr.	3.0	Tonifies Spleen; benefits Stomach
Sheng jiang	Ginger, fresh rhz.	3.0	Disperses cold; adjusts Nutritive Qi

Cautions in Use: Use carefully in people with low blood pressure.

49. Tang Gui and Gardenia Formula 温 清 飲

Common Usages: For eczema, dermatitis, tinea, and other skin conditions with associated symptoms of dry, dark skin, severe itching, ulcerated mucous membranes, and bleeding at site. Also used for uterine bleeding and excessive menstruation.

Traditional Usages and Functions: For heat conditions due to deficiency. Clears heat; cools and activates Blood; disperses stagnant Blood.

English Transliteration: Tang Gui and Gardenia Formula

Pinyin Mandarin Name: *Wen Qing Yin*

Forms Used: May be made into a tea or used in granular form.

Pinyin Name	Common English Name	Quantity in grams	Traditional Herb Function
Tang gui	Angelica, rt.	4.0	Tonifies and invigorates Blood
Shu di huang	Rehmannia (steamed)	4.0	Tonifies Liver and Kidneys; nourishes yin
Bai shao	Peony Alba, rx.	3.0	Pacifies Liver; tonifies Blood; preserves yin
Chuan xiang	Ligusticum, rhz.	3.0	Invigorates Blood; moves Qi
Huang lian	Coptis, rhz.	1.5	Clears heat; drains dampness
Huang qin	Scutellaria, rx.	3.0	Clears heat; drains damp heat
Huang bai	Phellodendron, bk.	1.5	Drains damp heat; quells Kidney fire
Zhi zi	Gardenia, fr.	2.0	Drains damp heat; cools Blood

Cautions in Use: Not to be used in people with a true cold condition.

50. Tang Gui and Ginseng Eight (Women's Precious Pills)　八珍湯

Common Usages: Frequently used for chronic fatigue syndrome with symptoms of overall fatigue; poor appetite and digestion; pale skin; dizziness; shortness of breath; and heart palpitations. Also used for irregular or deficient menstruation; and after childbirth, surgery, blood-loss trauma, and major illness.

Traditional Usages and Functions: Tonifies Qi and nourishes Blood.

English Transliteration: Tang Gui and Ginseng Eight or Women's Precious Pills

Pinyin Mandarin Name: *Ba Zhen Tang*

Forms Used: May be made into a tea or used in patent or granular forms.

Pinyin Name	Common English Name	Quantity in grams	Traditional Herb Function
Di Huang	Rehmannia (steamed)	3.0	Tonifies Liver and Kidneys; nourishes yin
Tang gui	Angelica, rt.	3.0	Tonifies and invigorates Blood
Fu ling	Poria (fungus)	3.0	Strengthens Spleen; moves dampness
Bai shao	Peony Alba, rx.	3.0	Pacifies Liver; tonifies Blood; preserves yin
Bai zhu	Atractylodes, rhz.	3.0	Tonifies Spleen Qi; dries dampness
Chuan xiang	Ligusticum, rhz.	2.0-3.0	Invigorates Blood; moves Qi
Ren shen	Ginseng, rx.	2.0-3.0	Tonifies Qi and Stomach; strengthens Spleen
Gan cao	Licorice, rx.	1.5	Tonifies Spleen; benefits Qi

Cautions in Use: Do not use at the onset of a cold or flu; may be used once recovery has begun.

51. Tang Gui and Indigo Formula　千金止帶丸

Common Usages: For vaginal infections with discharge (leukorrhea) and symptoms of fatigue, abdominal distension, poor appetitie, lower-back pain, and sore legs. Also used to treat trichomonas and other vaginal infections with discharge in the absence of accompanying symptoms; and the discharge, irritation, and/or yeast infections associated with the use of antibiotics and birth-control pills.

Traditional Usages and Functions: Tonifies Kidneys, Blood, and Uterus. Detoxifies and clears heat and dampness.

English Transliteration: Thousand Pieces of Gold Stop Leukorrhea Pill

Pinyin Mandarin Name: *Chien Chin Chih Tai Wan*

Forms Used: May be made into a tea or used in patent form.

Pinyin Name	Common English Name	Quantity in grams	Traditional Herb Function
Qing dai	Indigo, pigment	3.0	Clears damp heat
Dang shen	Codonopsis, rt.	2.5	Strengthens Qi; nourishes fluids
Mu li	Oyster Shell	2.5	Benefits yin; prevents leakage of fluids
Mu xiang	Saussurea, rt.	1.0	Moves and regulates Qi; strengthens Spleen
Tang gui	Angelica, rt.	1.0	Tonifies and invigorates Blood
Yan hu suo	Corydalis, rhz.	1.0	Moves Blood and Qi; alleviates pain
Xu duan	Dipsacus, rt.	1.0	Tonifies Liver and Kidneys; stops leukorrhea
Bai zhu	Atractylodes, rhz.	0.5	Tonifies Spleen Qi; dries dampness
Xiao hui xiang	Fennel, sd.	0.5	Regulates Qi; alleviates pain

Cautions in Use: Use carefully during pregnancy.

52. Tang Gui Four   四物湯

Common Usages: For irregular menstruation; threatened miscarriage; postbirth weakness; insufficient breast milk; and infertility. May also be used for dry skin; anemia; headaches; and select cases of lower-limb motor paralysis. Most often used for chronic conditions that are not severe.

Traditional Usages and Functions: Tonifies and activates Blood; regulates Liver; regulates menstruation.

English Transliteration: Tang Gui Four
Pinyin Mandarin Name: *Si Wu Tang*
Forms Used: May be made into a tea or used in patent or granular form.

Pinyin Name	Common English Name	Quantity in grams	Traditional Herb Function
Tang gui	Angelica, rt.	4.0	Tonifies and invigorates Blood
Shu di huang	Rehmannia (steamed)	4.0	Tonifies Liver and Kidneys; nourishes yin
Bai shao	Peony Alba, rx.	4.0	Tonifies Blood; preserves yin
Chuan xiang	Ligusticum, rhz.	2.0	Invigorates Blood; moves Qi

Cautions in Use: Unless combined with other herbs, Tang Gui Four should not be used for heavy blood loss following birth, for weak Spleen yang, or in the presence of diarrhea.

53. Tian Qi and Eucommia Formula　田七杜仲片

Common Usages: For chronic muscular, ligament, or arthritic pain with stiffness or swelling; chronic low back pain and knee weakness. Particularly effective for the back pain associated with movements such as bending and lifting.

Traditional Usages and Functions: For Kidney deficiency associated with slip-fall injuries. Tonifies Kidneys, moves Blood, and alleviates pain.

English Transliteration: Tian Qi and Eucommia Formula
Pinyin Mandarin Name: *Tin Tzat To Chung* Pills
Forms Used: May be made into a tea or used in patent form.

Pinyin Name	Common English Name	Quantity in grams	Traditional Herb Function
Tian qi	Pseudoginseng, rt.	6.0	Reduces swelling; alleviates pain; moves Blood stagnation
Du zhong	Eucommia, bk.	5.0	Tonifies Liver and Kidneys; strengthens sinews and bones
Ren shen	Ginseng, rx.	2.5	Tonifies Original Qi; strengthens Spleen

Pinyin Name	Common English Name	Quantity in grams	Traditional Herb Function
Lu rong	Cornu Cervi	2.0	Benefits Essence and Blood; strengthens sinews and bones
Rou gui	Cinnamon, rx.	1.0	Warms Kidney yang
Ru xiang	Frankincense, gum	3.0	Invigorates Blood; alleviates pain; promotes healing
Sang ji sheng	Loranthus, hb.	3.0	Tonifies Liver and Kidneys; expels damp
Hu gu	Panthera T.	3.5	Strengthens sinews and bones
Du huo	Angelica du huo (yellow), rt.	3.0	Expels wind damp; alleviates pain

Cautions in Use: Do not use during pregnancy.

54. Tu-Huo and Loranthus Formula　　獨活寄生湯

Common Usages: Used most often for chronic lower-back pain or rheumatic sciatica. Also used for chronic arthritis accompanied by chills, pain in lower back and knees, difficulty stretching legs, and/or severe numbness and spasms with pain.

Traditional Usages and Functions: Dispels wind and damp; tonifies Qi and Blood; strengthens Liver and Kidneys; relieves spasmodic pain.

English Transliteration: Tu-Huo and Loranthus

Pinyin Mandarin Name: *Du Huo Ji Sheng Tang*

Forms Used: May be made into a tea or used in patent and granular forms.

Pinyin Name	Common English Name	Quantity in grams	Traditional Herb Function
Du huo	Angelica du huo (yellow), rt.	4.5	Expels wind damp; alleviates pain
Qin jiao	Gentian, rt.	4.5	Expels wind damp
Fang feng	Siler, rt.	4.5	Expels wind dampness; alleviates pain
Xi xin	Asarum, hb.	4.5	Expels wind; disperses cold; alleviates pain

Pinyin Name	Common English Name	Quantity in grams	Traditional Herb Function
Rou gui	Cinnamon, rx.	4.5	Warms Kidney yang; warms up Blood
Sang ji sheng	Loranthus, hb.	4.5	Tonifies Liver and Kidneys; expels damp
Du zhong	Eucommia, bk.	4.5	Tonifies Liver and Kidneys; strengthens sinews and bones
Shu di huang	Rehmannia (steamed)	3.0	Tonifies Blood; nourishes yin
Niu xi	Achyranthes, rt.	4.5	Strengthens sinews and bones; benefits joints
Tang gui	Angelica, rt.	3.0	Tonifies and invigorates Blood
Bai shao	Peony Alba, rx.	3.0	Pacifies Liver; tonifies Blood; preserves yin
Chuan xiang	Ligusticum, rhz.	4.5	Invigorates Blood; moves Qi
Ren shen	Ginseng, rx.	4.5	Tonifies Original Qi; strengthens Spleen
Fu ling	Poria (fungus)	4.5	Strengthens Spleen
Gan cao	Licorice, rx.	3.0	Tonifies Qi; harmonizes other herbs

Cautions in Use: Do not use during pregnancy.

55. Xanthium and Magnolia Formula 鼻炎片

Common Usages: For pain associated with severe sinus infections accompanied by yellow phlegm and thick, foul-smelling discharge. Also used for mild allergy and hay-fever symptoms including runny nose and congestion in face.

Traditional Usages and Functions: For heat conditions associated with severe sinus infections. Dispels wind heat and opens nasal passages.

English Transliteration: Xanthium and Magnolia Formula

Pinyin Mandarin Name: *Bi Yan Pian*

Forms Used: May be made into a tea or used in patent form.

Pinyin Name	Common English Name	Quantity in grams	Traditional Herb Function
Xin yi hua	Magnolia, fl.	5.0	Expels wind; opens nasal passages
Cang er zi	Xanthium, fl.	4.5	Opens nasal passages; expels dampness
Huang bai	Phellodendron, bk.	1.5	Drains damp heat; detoxifies fire poison
Gan cao	Licorice, rx.	1.5	Moistens Lungs; stops coughing; harmonizes other herbs
Jie geng	Platycodon, rt.	1.0	Circulates Lung Qi; expels phlegm
Wu wei zi	Schisandra, fr.	1.0	Contains leakage of Lung Qi; stops cough
Lian qiao	Forsythia, fr.	1.5	Expels externally contracted wind heat
Bai zhi	Angelica, rt.	1.5	Expels wind; opens nasal passages
Zhi mu	Anemarrhenae, rhz.	1.0	Nourishes yin; moistens dryness; clears heat
Ye ju hua	Chrysanthemum, Wild	1.5	Quells fire; detoxifies fire poison
Fang feng	Siler, rt.	1.0	Expels wind dampness; alleviates pain
Jing jie	Schizonepeta, hb.	1.0	Releases exterior; expels itch brought on by exposure to wind

Cautions in Use: None.

CHAPTER EIGHT

Treating 25 Common Ailments with Herbal Formulas

Introduction

This chapter contains in-depth discussions of twenty-five of the most common ailments experienced by individuals and treated by practitioners, describing symptoms in detail in both traditional Oriental Medicine terms and conventional medical language. It also includes recommendations of specific formulas, all of them found in this book. According to the comprehensive and sophisticated diagnostic and treatment systems of Oriental Medicine, common ailments such as acne, arthritis, constipation, and high blood pressure, to name just a few, are never viewed as static conditions, with one set of clear-cut symptoms that are the same for everyone. Rather, they are seen as being caused by one or more particular *patterns* of imbalance, each of which has a specific set of symptoms that requires a specific herbal formula. Back pain, for example, in our discussion, may be caused by any one of eight different imbalances—wind cold, wind damp, and deficient Kidney Yin among them—each of which requires a different herbal remedy.

When we offer you a choice of two or more formulas, it will be useful to go back to Chapter Seven and reread the entries for those formulas. In that way, you can choose the formula most appropriate for your circumstances and state of health. For example, you may want to use a formula that not only treats your ailment, but also has a tonifying or a Blood-circulating effect.

When we suggest using a combination of formulas to treat an ailment, we mean that you literally may take the formulas together and at the same time. Since many of these formulas are available as patent medications—and therefore come in pill or tablet form—taking two formulas together is easy. Where you have prepared your own formulas in liquid form, the two preparations may be combined and cooked in the same container and then taken as needed.

For each ailment or imbalance, we recommend the most appropriate and effective formulas that are featured in this book. It's important to note, however, that there are thousands of Chinese herbal formulas, many of which are excellent—and sometimes even more appropriate— treatment choices. That is why we always strongly recommend that you work with a qualified practitioner, particularly in the case of serious or chronic ailments. He or she can monitor your recovery, make the most appropriate recommendations for herbal treatment, and adjust formulas to your specific needs.

Acne

Acne is a skin disease with many causes. While the most common causes are dietary and emotional, skin disorders are often the result of more complex patterns of imbalance. Due to the complexity of skin disorders, the wide range of their symptoms, and the differences in the herbal formulas used to treat them, care must be taken to make the correct diagnosis and choose the proper formula.

If you don't experience relief of some sort within a few days, please consult with a practitioner who is familiar with treating the skin. Formulas often must be carefully adjusted for the individual to get significant results.

Acne Imbalances

- Lung-heat acne patterns frequently occur on the forehead and around the nose as whiteheads and blackheads showing as raised, reddened areas that are only slightly itchy. Other Lung-heat symptoms may include dry stools, a sense of dryness in the mouth and throat, and a reddish tongue. The formula most likely to help this acne pattern is **Lonicera and Forsythia,** but you may want to contact your practitioner for a more specific formulation.

- Stomach-heat acne patterns show as blackheads and whiteheads with raised, red areas, usually around the mouth and on the chest and upper back. Other symptoms of this pattern include an oily face, large appetite with little or no weight gain, dry mouth and bad breath, dry stools, a preference for cold drinks, and a red tongue. The formula most useful in treating this acne pattern is **Tang Gui and Gardenia.**

- Blood-heat acne patterns affect the area around the nose and mouth, and between the eyebrows, showing as raised, red areas. Along with this raised, red area, facial flushing often accompanies certain emotions or exposure to heat. Premenstrual women see an increase in symptoms. Other symptoms of this pattern include dry stools, yellow urine, and a red tongue tip. The formula most useful for this acne pattern is **Tang Gui and Gardenia.**

- Heat-toxin acne patterns show most often on the upper back and chest, many times with inflamed and painful lesions. Often there is scarring after the lesions heal. General symptoms of this pattern include constipation or dry stools, and a red tongue with a dry coat. The best formula for this pattern is **Gentiana.**

- Damp-toxin-with-blood-stasis acne patterns show as deep, inflamed, and painful cysts and nodules involving the whole face, neck, and back. The skin is usually oily, and often there is pitted scarring. Other symptoms may include headaches, a purple tongue with a coat, and a feeling of toxicity. The best formula to use is **Gentiana.**

Alcohol and Drug Abuse (Also Depression and Mania)

Drug abuse, no matter what form it takes, is best treated with a combination of counseling, herbs, and acupuncture. Counseling is the major part of therapy, but herbal formulas can detoxify the body, provide a mild calming effect without sedation, and normalize and strengthen general health. Acupuncture provides similar therapeutic effects.

As everyone knows, excessive alcohol and drug use affects the liver. But alcohol and drug abuse also injures the Yin and raises false heat symptoms such as facial flushing, irritability, and headaches. Other symptoms may include spontaneous sweating, insomnia, and depression or hyperactivity.

Alcohol and Drug Abuse Imbalances

- Alcohol and drug abuse is often accompanied by patterns of mental and emotional imbalance. Symptoms of these imbalances include moodiness, restlessness, sadness with a desire to cry, insomnia, anger, sighing, and a tongue with a thin, white coat. In Oriental Medicine, the Heart is said to store the Spirit. Therefore, one of the formulas recommended for treating substance abuse contains two major herbs that are renowned for their therapeutic affect on the Heart and Liver. The formula used is **Bupleurum and Dragon Bone**.

- Substance abuse accompanied by a deficiency of the Heart and Spleen may include symptoms of excessive thinking, a tendency to mania, palpitations, insomnia, dizziness, a pale face, fatigue, poor appetite, and a pale tongue with a thin, white coat. A good formula choice for treatment would be **Ginseng and Longan**. If there is also diarrhea, you may use **Ginseng and Atractylodes**.

- With Liver Qi stagnation, symptoms may include depression, belching, emotional instability, poor appetite, possible vomiting, a sensation of fullness in the stomach or abdomen, a thin, greasy coating on the tongue, and frequent sighing. The formula of choice would be **Bupleurum and Tang Gui**.

- With Qi stagnation combined with fire, symptoms include restlessness, constipation, reddened eyes, headache, a dry mouth, irritability with "quick anger," acid regurgitation, ringing in the ears, a bitter taste in the mouth, and a red tongue. The best formula might be **Gentiana**.

- The last alcohol-and-drug-abuse pattern is due to a Yin deficiency leading to strong fire, and includes symptoms such as palpitations, dizziness, sore or weak lower back, depression, quick anger, restlessness, insomnia, and a red tongue. The formulas of choice would be **Ginseng and Zizyphus** or **Concha Marguerita and Ligustrum**.

Allergies

Allergies are either seasonal, such as hay fever, or constant, such as allergic rhinitis. Both patterns include symptoms of nasal congestion or runny nose, possible headache or loss of smell, itching of the eyes and/or nose, and a general loss of energy.

Allergy Imbalances

- Wind-cold allergy patterns include symptoms of clear, profuse nasal discharge, a loss of smell, possibly a headache with an aversion to cold, and itching and sneezing—especially when seasonal. A good formula to choose for this pattern would be **Ma Huang**.
- Wind-heat allergy patterns include symptoms of fever, nasal congestion with yellow and sometimes malodorous phlegm, a loss of smell, and a thin, yellow coat on the tongue. These symptoms call for **Xanthium and Magnolia**.
- Wind-cold allergy patterns accompanied by internal Yang deficiency will include symptoms of cold intolerance, a runny nose with copious, clear phlegm, a headache or sensation of heaviness in the head or body, swelling in the neck and face, possible cough from postnasal phlegm, fatigue, shortness of breath, little or no perspiration with a mild fever, and a pale tongue with a white coat. The best formula for this allergy pattern is **Rehmannia Eight**.

Note: Always take into consideration that someone who is strongly allergic may be allergic to one or more of the herbs in the formula.

Arthritis

In Oriental Medicine, arthritis is viewed as an obstruction of Qi and Blood circulation. This is usually caused by an invasion of wind, cold, and dampness due to a weakness in the Protective Qi, or a body's predisposition to obstruction, or repeated exposure to either wind, cold, or dampness that creates an environment that allows obstruction to develop. In Oriental Medicine, the characteristic joint pain and stiffness of arthritis is called *Bi*, the term used to describe the various arthritis imbalances, which are grouped according to clusters of symptoms.

Arthritis Imbalances

- Wandering Bi includes symptoms of pain that move from one joint to the other, with stiff or limited joint movements, and possible wind-heat or wind-cold symptoms such as an aversion to wind or drafts. The treatment of choice would be a combination of **Clematis and Stephania** and **Corydalis Tuber**. Another good formula for this pattern of imbalance is the **Pueraria Combination**.

- Fixed Bi includes symptoms of painful, swollen joints with a heavy sensation and a fixed location of the pain, which worsens with cold and damp, a sense of numbness in the muscle around the joints, limited range of motion, and a white, greasy coat on the tongue. **Qiang-Huo and Turmeric**, **Stephania and Astragalus**, and **Tu-Huo and Loranthus** are the best formulas used for this pattern of imbalance.
- Painful Bi includes symptoms of fixed pain with no redness or swelling, very painful joints that are aggravated by cold and limited in movement, possible sensation of heat when movement is attempted, and a white coat on the tongue. The best formula for this pattern of imbalance is **Qiang-Huo and Turmeric**, to which **Corydalis Tuber** may be added to enhance pain relief.
- Febrile Bi includes symptoms of heavy, swollen, and painful joints accompanied by redness and sensitivity to touch, and pain with all movements. Pain may be relieved with cool or cold compresses. The pain of Febrile Bi may also move from joint to joint, but unlike Wandering Bi, the pain of Febrile Bi is more likely to manifest in one joint at a time, often with symptoms of wind-heat such as fever, perspiration, thirst, restlessness, an aversion to wind and drafts, and a dry, yellow coat on the tongue. The best treatment choice is **Clematis and Stephania**.
- Deficient Qi and Blood Bi usually include symptoms of chronic swollen, painful, and deformed joints that severely limit physical activity, numbness in the extremities with contraction, fatigue, shortness of breath, blurred vision, loose stools, dizziness, poor appetite, and a pale tongue with a thin, white coat. The treatment of choice is a combination of **Qiang-Huo and Turmeric** and **Tang Gui and Ginseng Eight**.
- Deficient Kidney Yin or Yang Bi includes symptoms of chronic joint pain with deformity of the joints, pale tissue, local swelling and contraction, worsening of pain at night, fatigue, sore and weak lower back, leukorrhea or sperm leakage, and blurred vision. In the case of deficient Kidney Yin, there will be a thin, red tongue with no coat. In the case of deficient Kidney Yang, there will be a pale and swollen tongue with a white coat. The best formula where there is deficient Kidney Yin is **Anemarrhena, Phellodendron, and Rehmannia**. Where there is deficient Kidney Yang, the best choice is **Tu-Huo and Loranthus**.

Asthma

It is important to recognize that treating asthma is a complex and difficult road to travel, whether using natural or biochemical remedies. Results are rarely rapid, but they can be achieved with patience and awareness.

It is best to work with a practitioner when treating this disorder. Also let your conventional physician know what you are doing so that he can adjust your conventional medications accordingly. As with any other chronic disorder, the longer you have had the problem, and the more conventional medications you are on, the longer it will take to work your way off of them. This is where it is important to have your conventional practitioner monitor your progress and work with your dosage. Your practitioner should be more than willing to help you reduce dosages of conventional drugs, since, more than anyone else, conventional physicians realize the long-term effects of such medications.

Asthma Imbalances

- Wind-cold asthma patterns include symptoms of breathlessness, a sensation of fullness in the chest, cough with profuse, white, watery sputum, no perspiration, headache, discomfort when even slightly cold, and a thin, white coat on the tongue. A good formula for this pattern is **Ma Huang**.
- Wind-heat asthma patterns include symptoms of breathlessness, shortness of breath, yellow sticky phlegm, restlessness and irritability, intolerance to drafts, fever and sweating, a sensation of fullness in the chest, and a thin, yellow coat on the tongue. The best formula to treat this pattern is **Apricot and Fritillaria**.
- Asthma patterns characterized by phlegm that interferes with Lung Qi include symptoms of profuse and sticky sputum, a sensation of fullness in the chest, nausea with poor appetite, shortness of breath, coughing, poor digestion and metabolism, loss of sense of taste, and a white, greasy-looking coat on the tongue. The best formula for this group of symptoms is **Citrus and Pinellia**.
- Asthma patterns characterized by stagnant Qi that interferes with Lung Qi include symptoms of emotional instability with depression and anxiety, sudden loss of breath, discomfort in the throat (a feeling of having something lodged there), chest pain with a sensation of fullness in chest, insomnia, palpitations, and a thin coat

on the tongue. This asthma pattern is more acute and may require more than home care. The best formula for this set of symptoms is **Cyperus and Ligusticum**.

- Deficiency-of-Lung-Qi asthma patterns include symptoms of shortness of breath, fatigue, aversion to drafts, difficulty speaking due to fatigue, spontaneous sweating, a dry mouth, flushed face, and a light red tongue. A good formula for these symptoms is **Ginseng and Astragalus**.

- With deficiency-of-Lung-Yin asthma patterns, the person has a chronic asthma condition with shortness of breath, sticky, scanty sputum, a dry throat, night sweats, a red, dry tongue, and an emaciated look. These symptoms are often seen in people who have been taking asthma medication to dry up phlegm for a long time. With these symptoms, it is especially important to work with a practitioner. The best formula for treating this group of symptoms is the **Fritillaria Extract Tablet**.

- Deficiency-of-Spleen-Qi asthma patterns include symptoms of shortness of breath, coughing with copious sputum, fatigue, poor appetite, diarrhea or frequent loose stools, and a pale tongue with a greasy or white coat. The formula of choice is **Ginseng and Atractylodes**.

- Deficiency-of-Kidney-Qi asthma patterns include symptoms of chronic asthma with shortness of breath, difficulty inhaling completely, fatigue that worsens with exertion, easy perspiration, cold extremities, an emaciated look, and a pale tongue. The best formula for this group of symptoms is **Rehmannia Eight**.

Back Pain

Back pain—one of the most common ailments in our society—can be caused by a sudden injury, by repeated stresses to the back, or by an imbalance within the body that predisposes the back to injury when combined with either sudden or excessive movement or lifting.

Back Pain Imbalances

- Back pain caused by cold-damp imbalances includes symptoms of coldness and pain in the lower back, difficulty moving (as if back were semifrozen), pain that worsens and is aggravated by lying down or by climatic conditions such as rain, and a white, greasy coat on the tongue. The best formula for this pattern of back pain is **Tu-Huo and Loranthus**.

- Back pain caused by heat-damp imbalances includes symptoms of pain in the lower back with a sensation of localized heat that is aggravated by climatic heat and improves with movement, swollen extremities, restlessness, a strong thirst, scant, yellow urine, and a yellow, greasy coat on the tongue. Good formulas for this pattern of back pain are **Anemarrhena, Phellodendron, and Rehmannia** and **Gentiana**.

- Back pain caused by wind-cold imbalances includes symptoms of a cold feeling in the lower back that improves with hot compresses, often accompanied by fever and an aversion to cold, pain that often radiates down into the legs or up into the mid-back, and a thin, white coat on the tongue. Two formulas that are good for this pattern of back pain are **Tu-Huo and Loranthus** and **Rehmannia Eight**.

- Back pain caused by wind-damp imbalances includes symptoms of sore, heavy or painful lower back, difficulty stretching, fever with an aversion to wind or chills, possible edema in the face and extremities, and a greasy coat on the tongue. The best formula for this pattern of back pain is **Tu-Huo and Loranthus**.

- Back pain caused by injury includes symptoms of pain on movement, sudden onset of pain, pain on specific movements such as leg raises, and sensitivity to touch. The best formula for back pain caused by injury is **Tian Ma and Eucommia**.

- Back pain caused by deficient Kidney Yin includes symptoms of aching and weak lower back, weak knees, strong thirst, pain that worsens on exertion, a sensation of heat in the palms and soles, and a reddish tongue. The best formula for this pattern of back pain is **Rehmannia Six**.

- Back pain caused by deficient Kidney Yang includes symptoms of back pain that worsens with cold weather and drafts, difficulty getting warm, cold extremities, pale face, slow movements, and a pale tongue with a white coat. The formula of choice for this pattern of back pain is **Rehmannia Eight**.

- Back pain caused by wind-cold-damp imbalances includes symptoms of a cold feeling in the lower back that improves with hot compresses, often accompanied by a fever and an aversion to cold and wind (drafts), pain that often radiates down into the legs or up into the mid-back, a sore, heavy or painful lower back accompanied by difficulty in stretching, possible edema in the face and extremities, and a greasy coating on the tongue. The best formula for this pattern of imbalance is **Tu-Huo and Loranthus**.

Common Cold or Flu

Symptoms of the common cold are often masked, or simply ignored, by the use of over-the-counter remedies or prescribed antibiotics. But such treatment increases the chance of having the virus or bacteria penetrate deeper into the body, only to show up later as bronchitis or asthma.

The common-cold and flu patterns described below will help you choose the best herbal formula for throwing off a cold or flu quickly and completely so that you are not suffering with cold or flu symptoms for weeks or months afterward. This latter pattern weakens the body's self-protective ability and can allow an illness to move to progressively deeper levels within the body, later expressing itself as more chronic or extreme symptoms.

Common Cold or Flu Imbalances

- Wind-cold patterns of common cold or flu include symptoms of fever with an aversion to cold and an inability to feel warm no matter how many blankets one uses, a headache with a feeling of tightness, heaviness, or a dull ache, nasal congestion or a runny nose with clear phlegm, sneezing, a sore throat, little or no sweating, a cough with thin, white or clear sputum, and a thin, white coat on the tongue. The formula that is most useful for treating these symptoms is Ma Huang.
- Wind-heat patterns of common cold or flu include symptoms of fever with an aversion to drafts, headache, sweating, nasal congestion, sore throat, dry mouth, strong thirst, especially for cold drinks, sticky yellow sputum, and a thin yellow coat on the tongue. The best formulas for these symptoms are **Lonicera and Forsythia** or **Ilex and Evodia**.
- Colds accompanied by strong deficiency signs, such as the inability to speak clearly or strongly, a serious aversion to cold accompanied by an inability to warm up, a pale tongue and face, and general body aches, should be assessed by a practitioner due to the

complexity of the symptoms and the need to adjust formulations. A formula that can be used for these symptoms is **Ginseng and Astragalus**.

Constipation

Constipation is generally regarded simply as difficulty in moving bowels. But using herbs or drugs merely to "force" a stool movement can in reality create an addiction in the body for stronger and stronger laxatives.

The goal in treating constipation, therefore, is to normalize bowel function and allow the person to release stools naturally without herbs or medications. This becomes more difficult with advanced age and overuse of laxatives, but it is not impossible. Diet must also be addressed. For example, a person with internal heat must reduce their intake of spicy foods and alcohol.

Constipation Imbalances

- Internal-heat constipation patterns include symptoms of dry and hard feces, scanty, dark yellow urine, a flushed complexion, a sensation of heat in the body all the time, strong thirst, especially for cold fluids, bad breath, restlessness, and a sensation of fullness and pain in the abdomen, many times combined with a reddish tongue, usually with a yellow coat. A good formula for this group of symptoms is **Apricot Seed and Linum**.
- Stagnant Qi constipation patterns include symptoms of difficulty in releasing stool, even with a strong urge to do so, fullness and pain in the abdomen, poor appetite, belching, and a thin, greasy coat on the tongue. Good formulas for this group of symptoms are **Bupleurum and Tang Gui** and **Cimicafuga**.
- Qi-deficiency constipation patterns include symptoms of normal stool relative to consistency and moisture, but difficulty in releasing stool normally. Many times there will be sweating, and possibly shortness of breath, during and after trying to pass stool, along with a pale complexion, fatigue, weakness in the extremities, and a pale tongue with a white coat. The best formula for these symptoms is **Ginseng and Astragalus**.
- Blood-deficiency constipation patterns include symptoms of dizziness, a pale, lusterless complexion, pale lips and tongue, pal-

pitations, and blurred vision. Generally, a good formula for these symptoms is **Tang Gui Four**.

- Yang-deficiency constipation patterns include symptoms of excessive urination, pale complexion, cold extremities, difficulty getting warm, achiness or weakness in lower back, cold sensation in the abdomen and spine, and a pale tongue with a white coat. One of the best formulas for these symptoms is **Rehmannia Eight**.
- For constipation in the elderly due to yin deficiency, **Polygonum Multiflorum** alone may be used daily.
- For constipation that occurs after the use of excessive amounts of alcohol and/or spicy foods, with accompanying symptoms of a red flushed face, irritability, and insomnia, a good formula to use is **Bupleurum and Dragon Bone**.

Cough

Coughing can have many causes beyond those covered in this book, and a cough that lasts beyond a few days should be seen by a practitioner for more specific treatment.

Cough Imbalances

- Wind-cold coughs include symptoms of thin, white phlegm, mild fever, an aversion to drafts or cold, headache, nasal congestion, possible runny nose with thin, clear or white phlegm, sometimes soreness throughout the body, no perspiration, and a thin, white tongue coating. The best formula for these symptoms is **Ma Huang**.
- Wind-heat coughs include symptoms of thick, yellow phlegm, strong thirst, especially for cold fluids, aversion to drafts, sweating, headache, dry and sore throat, and a thin, yellow coat on the tongue. The best formula to use for these symptoms is **Lonicera and Forsythia**.
- Dry-heat coughs include symptoms of little or no phlegm, or scant phlegm tinged with blood, dry throat and mouth, preference for cold drinks, aversion to drafts, possible fever, and red tongue. The formula of choice would be **Fritillaria Extract Tablet**.
- Damp-phlegm coughs include symptoms of copious watery and possibly foamy phlegm, a sensation of fullness in the chest, poor

appetite, loose stools, fatigue, and a white, greasy-looking coat on the tongue. Two formulas good for these symptoms are **Citrus and Pinellia** and **Major Six Herbs**.

- Flaming Liver fire coughs include symptoms of coughing accompanied by a painful sensation under the ribs on the right side, coughing that worsens with emotional changes, dry throat, flushed face, and a dry, thin, yellow coat on the tongue. The formula of choice would be **Gentiana**.
- Chronic coughs due to Yin deficiency of the Lungs include symptoms of dry, scanty, or bloody sputum, or vomiting of blood, dry mouth and throat, afternoon fevers, flushed cheeks, heat sensations in the palms and feet, insomnia, fatigue, night sweating, and a red tongue. A good formula for these symptoms is **Rehmannia Six**.
- Chronic coughs due to Qi deficiency of the Lungs include symptoms of a weakened voice, shortness of breath, fatigue, an aversion to drafts, spontaneous sweating, discomfort in the throat, and a dry mouth. A good formula for this set of symptoms is **Ginseng and Astragalus**.

Diarrhea

In cases of diarrhea, drink plenty of fluids and be careful not to get dehydrated. If symptoms do not clear up fairly rapidly, consult with a practitioner.

Diarrhea Imbalances

- Wind-cold and/or -damp diarrhea patterns include symptoms of watery diarrhea with gurgling and pain in the abdomen, vomiting, possible fever, aversion to drafts, nasal congestion, headache, and a thin, white or greasy-looking coat on the tongue. A good formula for these symptoms is **Agastache**.
- Damp-heat diarrhea patterns include symptoms of yellowish, smelly stools with abdominal pain and a burning sensation in the anus, scanty yellow or brownish urine, restlessness, a strong thirst for cold drinks, and a yellow, greasy-looking coat on the tongue. The formula of choice is **Gentiana**.
- Diarrhea caused by food stagnation in the stomach and intestine includes symptoms of abdominal pain and gurgling, smelly stool

with undigested food in it, acid regurgitation, foul-smelling phlegm, poor appetite, a sensation of fullness in the abdominal region, and a thick greasy coating on the tongue. A good formula for this group of symptoms is **Citrus and Pinellia**.

- Diarrhea caused by excessive Liver Qi attacking the Spleen includes symptoms of emotional instability and abdominal pain that worsens with emotional upsets such as depression, anger, or anxiety, burping, sometimes of acid, and little or no appetite. The formula of choice is **Bupleurum and Tang Gui**.

- Diarrhea caused by a deficiency of the Spleen and Stomach includes symptoms of loose or watery stool with food particles in it, diarrhea made worse by fatty or oily foods, a sensation of fullness in the abdomen, a pale, lusterless complexion, fatigue, poor appetite, and a pale tongue with a white coat. The two formulas most often used for these symptoms are **Ginseng and Atractylodes** and **Ginseng and Astragalus**.

- Diarrhea caused by deficient Kidney Yang includes symptoms of gurgling and pain in the abdomen and diarrhea that worsens at dawn, sometimes coming in several waves of loose stool, with abdominal cramping reduced after stool is released. Other symptoms include cold extremities, an inability to get warm, weak and sore lower back, and a pale tongue with a white coat. The best formula for these symptoms is **Rehmannia Eight**.

Dizziness and Vertigo

Dizziness and vertigo can be signs of dangerous illnesses, and it is important to see a qualified practitioner to rule out serious brain disease or tumor. Once that is done, however, herbal formulas can produce excellent results. Diet and lifestyle factors can worsen these conditions, and caffeine, chocolate, alcohol, nicotine, and certain foods should be avoided while under herbal treatment. If you don't see results in a few days, please consult with a practitioner.

Dizziness and Vertigo Imbalances

- Dizziness and vertigo caused by rising Liver Yang include symptoms of headache that is worsened by strong emotions such as frustration, anger, or bitterness, or by overwork, restlessness, a bitter taste in the mouth, and a red tongue with a yellow coat. Two formulas useful in treating these symptoms are **Bupleurum and Dragon Bone** and **Gentiana**.

- Dizziness and vertigo caused by deficient Kidney Essence is often seen in the elderly or in individuals, particularly men, who have indulged in excessive sexual activity, including excessive masturbation. The latter activity can deplete Kidney Essence and thus deprive the Brain of proper nourishment. Symptoms of this pattern of dizziness and vertigo include forgetfulness, ringing in the ears, a sore and weak lower back, and either cold extremities with a pale tongue and an inability to get warm (Kidney-Yang deficiency), or a red tongue with a sensation of heat in the palms and soles (Kidney-Yin deficiency). Where there is deficient Kidney Essence with accompanying Yang deficiency, use **Rehmannia Eight**. For deficient Kidney Essence with accompanying Yin deficiency, use **Rehmannia Six**.

- Dizziness and vertigo caused by deficient Qi and Blood often occurs after a major blood loss, long-term bleeding, or with chronic diseases involving impairment of the circulatory system. Often there is an accompanying imbalance of the Stomach or Spleen. Symptoms include pale skin, fingernail beds, and lips, insomnia, palpitations, fatigue, lethargy, little or no appetite, and a pale tongue with a thin coat. Several formulas are useful in treating this pattern of symptoms, including **Ginseng and Longan**, **Ginseng and Tang Gui Ten**, and **Ginseng and Astragalus**.

- Dizziness and vertigo caused by excessive thick phlegm obstructing the Spleen and Stomach includes symptoms of a sensation of heaviness in the head, fullness in the chest with a suffocating sensation, poor appetite, nausea, sleepiness, vomiting, and a white, greasy coating on the tongue. The formula of choice would be **Citrus and Pinellia**.

Ear Infections (Otitis)

Ear infections, especially in children, should first be checked out by a qualified pediatrician or traditional practitioner, particularly in acute cases, to rule out any possibility of permanent damage. Any of the herbal formulas below can then be used under the supervision of the practitioner.

Ear Infection Imbalances

- Acute ear infections caused by Liver and Gallbladder fire patterns include symptoms of earache, impaired hearing, a feeling of fullness in the head, ringing in the ears, fever and/or chills, sometimes sensitivity in the area of the skull behind the ear, and a red tongue with a white or yellow coat. A good choice for this pattern of acute ear infection is **Gentiana**.
- Chronic ear infections caused by deficiency-fire patterns include symptoms of repeated nose and throat infections preceding the ear infections, gradual hearing loss, ringing in the ears, sometimes vertigo, and a red tongue with little coating. Often, the individual's own voice sounds hollow to them when they speak. A good choice for this pattern of chronic ear infection is **Anemarrhena, Phellodendron, and Rehmannia**.

Gallstones

While an acute gallstone attack may sometimes require surgery, in most cases of gallstone imbalance there is sufficient early warning so that diet and lifestyle changes, combined with the correct herbal treatment, can successfully ward off a more severe condition. Herbal formulas are especially effective in treating early symptoms of gallstones, including burping, indigestion, occasional gallstone pain, and even mild jaundice (yellowing of the skin). Consultation with a qualified practitioner is strongly recommended to evaluate your condition properly, to assess whether surgery is necessary, and to monitor all aspects of treatment.

Gallstone Imbalances

- Gallstone imbalances caused by obstruction of the bile duct will often include symptoms of rapidly appearing jaundice, aversion to cold, rib pain on the right side that progresses to the shoulder and back, alternating chills and fever, a strong bitter taste in the mouth, nausea and vomiting, a dry throat, poor appetite, a sensation of fullness in the abdomen, pale gray or white stools, hot, scanty, and yellowish urine, and a red tongue with a thick, yellow coat. Several formulas may be used for this pattern, including

Minor Bupleurum, Rhubarb and Scutellaria, or **Bupleurum, Inula, and Cyperus**.

Hemorrhoids

Hemorrhoids are the result of stagnant Qi and Blood, and there are several causes for this disorder: excess dry-heat patterns of imbalance from overconsumption of fried, hot, and spicy foods and/or overconsumption of alcohol, sometimes combined with dampness, deficient yin, or stagnant Blood; lack of exercise; carrying heavy loads; sitting or standing for long periods of time; and chronic constipation. Often there is bright red blood, itching, or pain, depending on severity of the disorder.

Hemorrhoid Imbalances

- Where hemorrhoids are caused by an excess condition, symptoms will include bright red blood and sometimes profuse bleeding before and/or after bowel movement; a red tongue will also be present. The formula of choice for this pattern of hemorrhoids is **Cimicafuga**.
- Where hemorrhoids are caused by a deficiency condition, symptoms will include paler-colored blood, light bleeding, pale complexion, fatigue, dizziness, palpitations, insomnia, poor appetite, and a pale tongue. The choice of formula used for this pattern of hemorrhoids depends on other symptoms of excess or deficiency, and the advice of a practitioner is recommended. Several excellent formulas used to treat this pattern are **Ginseng and Tang Gui Ten**, **Ginseng and Longan**, **Ginseng and Astragalus**, **Tang Gui Four**, and **Apricot Seed and Linum**.

High Blood Pressure (Hypertension)

Hypertension, or high blood pressure, can be caused by one or more excess or deficiency imbalances, as described below. It is especially important to work with both your conventional practitioner and an Oriental Medicine practitioner to treat hypertension.

High Blood Pressure Imbalances

- Hypertension caused by excess Liver-fire conditions includes symptoms of dizziness, headache (sharp pain), ringing in the ears, bitter taste in the mouth, nausea, irritability, constipation, restlessness, nightmares, flushed face, and a red tongue with a yellow coat. Effective formulas for treating this pattern are **Prunella and Scutellaria**, **Gentiana**, and **Bupleurum and Dragon Bone**.

- Hypertension caused by deficient-Liver-fire conditions includes symptoms of dizziness, headache (dull pain), a sore and weak lower back, ringing in the ears, insomnia, restlessness, a sensation of heat in the palms and soles, forgetfulness, palpitations, night sweats, dry eyes, blurred vision, and a red tongue with a thin coat. Several formulas have proven excellent for treating this pattern. They include **Anemarrhena, Phellodendron, and Rehmannia**, **Rehmannia and Magnetitum**, and **Rehmannia and Dogwood Fruit**, or the **Eight Immortal Long Life Pill**, depending on other symptoms present.

- Hypertension caused by deficient Kidney Yin includes symptoms of tinnitis (ringing in the ears), palpitation, sore and weak lower back, shortness of breath, insomnia, nightmares, eyelid or other muscle twitching, and a pale or red tongue with a white coat. The formulas of choice for this pattern are **Rehmannia Six** and **Eight Immortal Long Life Pill**.

- Hypertension caused by deficiency Qi and Blood includes symptoms of dizziness, especially after exertion, pale skin, lips, and fingernail beds, palpitations, insomnia, poor appetite, and a pale tongue. Two excellent formulas for this pattern are **Tang Gui and Ginseng Eight** and **Ginseng and Longan**.

- Hypertension due to obstruction of phlegm and dampness includes symptoms of headache, dizziness, a sensation of heaviness and tightness in the head, a sensation of fullness in the chest, palpitations, poor appetite, vomiting of phlegm, and a white tongue with a greasy coating. The formula of choice for this pattern is **Citrus and Pinellia**.

Note: The **Leonuris and Achyranthes** formula may be used supplementally to enhance the effect of any of the above formulas.

Immune System

Treating the immune system has been a large part of Oriental Medicine for thousands of years; the English transliteration for such treatment is "supporting the normal, nurturing the root." Unlike conventional medicine, Oriental Medicine always recognized the need to support the normal—the immune *function*—and nurture the root—the immune *system*—through the use of immune-supporting-and-enhancing tonics. In our culture, we find it difficult to understand that our ability to stay strong, or pass on strong genes, changes as we age. Support of the immune system is an important part of our everyday health, and its relative strength is often decisive in our ability to resist disease and not have to rely on medications in order to remain healthy and active.

Some people need additional immune support from birth just to remain healthy enough to keep up with all the various imbalances with which they come in contact. Others can abuse their bodies and suffer no problems whatsoever. In many ways, this is a matter of fate. But it is conscious choice, not fate, that leads us to try herbs and other Oriental healing practices to make up for the deficiencies we are born with or acquire. That is why you are reading this book.

While the balanced interaction of all Organ systems is the true basis for proper immune function, actual treatment of the immune system revolves around three main Organs: the Kidneys, which govern the individual's base or root immune function, inherited in part from his ancestors; the Spleen, which governs the nutritional or normal metabolic system; and the Lungs, which govern Qi and normal immediate protection from outside invaders.

Immune System Tonics

- Kidney-tonic formulas build the individual's base of essential energy and strengthen the whole system, increasing longevity and helping to maintain a youthful appearance and physical ability while retaining clarity of thought. Kidney-tonic formulas include **Cerebral Tonic Pills**, **Eight Immortal Long Life Pills**, **Polygonum Tablets**, **Panax Ginseng Capsules**, and **Rehmannia Six**.
- Spleen-tonic formulas help the body carry out the normal metabolic functions of digestion at optimal levels, thus allowing it to break down raw substances into needed nutrients and make nutrients available to the system. Spleen-tonic formulas include **Gin-**

seng and Atractylodes, Major Six Herbs, Ginseng and Longan, and Ginseng and Tang Gui Ten.
- Lung-tonic formulas provide a protective barrier against the outside world and bring in Air Qi so it can mix with Nutritive Qi from the Spleen to feed the system. The Lungs control the Qi, which is the most active aspect of the body's immune system. Lung-tonic formulas include **Ginseng and Atractylodes, Major Four Herbs**, and **Panax Ginseng Capsules**.

Indigestion

Indigestion can signal a wide range of illnesses, from a mild dietary upset to a perforated ulcer. It is important to see a qualified practitioner to rule out any serious medical problems before you use an herbal formula. A practitioner may prescribe a symptom-specific formula that will be far more effective than the more general formulas listed in this book. When you have ruled out any serious medical conditions, however, the formulas listed below can be quite effective in relieving the symptoms they treat. If you do not experience relief within a week or so, please see a practitioner.

Indigestion Imbalances

- Indigestion caused by food stagnation includes symptoms of Stomach pain, a sensation of fullness in Stomach, burping of acid, no appetite, vomiting of undigested food with a feeling of relief after vomiting, difficult bowel movements, and a greasy coat on the tongue. A good formula for this pattern of indigestion is **Citrus and Pinellia**.
- Indigestion caused by stagnant Liver Qi includes symptoms of Stomach pain that extends to the ribs with a sensation of distension in the stomach, frequent burping of acid, difficult bowel movements, a worsening of symptoms in the presence of stress, and a thin, white coat on the tongue. The best formula for this pattern is **Bupleurum and Tang Gui**.
- Indigestion caused by stagnant Liver Qi with Stomach Heat includes symptoms of intense gastric pain with a burning sensation in the Stomach, nausea, irritability, restlessness, burping of acid, a dry mouth with a bitter taste, and a red tongue with

a yellow coat. Good choices for this pattern of indigestion include the **Bupleurum, Inula, and Cyperus** formula, the **Gentiana** formulas, and the **Peony and Licorice** formula.

- Indigestion caused by deficient Stomach Yin includes symptoms of chronic, dull pain in the stomach area, dry mouth and throat, strong thirst, dry and hard stools, and a red and dry tongue. The best formula for this pattern is often **Rehmannia Six**.

- Indigestion caused by Blood stasis in the Stomach includes symptoms of chronic Stomach pain with localized stabbing pain that worsens with pressure, and a dark or purple tongue. For this pattern, you may combine **Tang Gui Four** and **Peony and Licorice**. If the pain is severe, you may also take the **Corydalis Tuber** formula.

- Indigestion caused by deficient Spleen and Stomach with internal Cold includes symptoms of chronic Stomach pain with acid and water regurgitation, poor appetite, fatigue, cold extremities, loose stools, a sensation of relief when warmth and mild pressure are applied to the Stomach (with a hot water bottle, for example), and a pale tongue with a thin, white coat. Two excellent treatment choices for this pattern are **Ginseng and Longan** or **Ginseng and Atractylodes**.

- Indigestion caused by internal Cold attacking the Stomach includes symptoms of sudden Stomach pain, an aversion to any type of coldness, a desire for warm liquids, a sensation of relief when warmth and mild pressure are applied to the Stomach (with a hot water bottle, for example), and a thin coat on the tongue. For this pattern, we do not recommend the use of an herbal formula. Instead, use a hot water bottle on the stomach and drink some ginger tea.

Insomnia

Insomnia covers a wide range of sleep disorders, including poor quality of sleep due to nightmares, sudden wakefulness with an inability to fall back to sleep, restless or disturbed sleep, and the inability to fall asleep at all. Most times, emotional disturbances are at the root of this disorder, including excessive worry or rumination over a long period of time. Long-term emotional disturbances can in turn create physical imbalances that exacerbate insomnia. Very often, therefore, herbal treatment is supplemented with lifestyle counseling.

Insomnia Imbalances

- Insomnia caused by excess Liver Fire includes symptoms of irritability, restlessness, strong thirst (especially for alcohol), red eyes, a bitter taste in the mouth, constipation, strong-smelling yellow urine, and a red tongue with a yellow coat. A good choice for this pattern is **Gentiana**.
- Insomnia caused by excess Phlegm and rising Heat includes symptoms of copious sputum, a sensation of fullness in the chest, a sensation of heaviness and tightness in the head, poor appetite, burping of acid, vomiting, restlessness, a bitter taste in the mouth, and a yellow, greasy coat on the tongue. The formula of choice for this pattern is **Citrus and Pinellia**.
- Insomnia caused by rising Heart fire includes symptoms of waking at night with active dreams or nightmares, palpitations, heat in the soles and palms that worsens at night, ringing in the ears, night sweats, dizziness, forgetfulness, sore and weak lower back, and a dry mouth with a red, lightly coated tongue. Two good formulas for this pattern are **Ginseng and Zizyphus** and **Concha Marguerita and Ligustrum**.
- Insomnia caused by deficient Heart and Spleen includes symptoms of waking at night with active dreams or nightmares, palpitations, poor appetite, blurred vision, forgetfulness, fatigue, little or no taste, dizziness, pale skin with a dull look on the face, and a pale tongue with a thin coat. The best formulas for this pattern are **Ginseng and Tang Gui Ten** and **Ginseng and Longan**.
- Insomnia caused by Qi and Blood deficiencies of the Heart and Gallbladder includes symptoms of nightmares, palpitations, poor confidence, constant worrying, a tendency to be easily frightened, frequent and excessive urination, shortness of breath, and a pale tongue. The best formulas for this pattern are **Ginseng and Zizyphus** and **Concha Marguerita and Ligustrum**.

Menopause

Menopause is often a normal and smooth life transition. Many times, however, it is accompanied by symptoms that are the result of complex imbalances, some of which have their origin in the use of birth-control pills or other drugs, and/or may be the result of prior surgeries. These symptoms are often both physical and mental, and in extreme cases can even be life threatening. If you don't experience relief from your symptoms within a few cycles, please consult a qualified practitioner.

Menopause Imbalances

- Menopausal symptoms caused by Liver stagnation and Spleen deficiency include symptoms of increasingly irregular menstruation, emotional imbalances such as depression, crying, melancholy, irritability, and mild paranoialike suspicions, a sensation of a fruit pit stuck in the throat, headaches, occasionally vertigo, loose stools, poor appetite, a sensation of heaviness or pain in the ribs, and a reddish tongue that may have a thin coat. Excellent formulas for this pattern are **Bupleurum and Tang Gui** and **Angelica** used in combination, **Cyperus and Ligusticum,** or **Bupleurum and Dragon Bone**.
- Menopausal symptoms caused by deficient Kidney Yin include irregular menses, blurred vision, dizziness, insomnia, excessive dreaming, hair loss, failing memory, hot flashes, especially of the palms and soles, sore and weak lower back and knees, strong thirst, constipation, scanty yellow urination, and a red tongue with a thin coat. The formulas of choice fo this pattern include **Rehmannia Six** and **Anemarrhena, Phellodendron, and Rehmannia**. With hair loss, include the **Polygonum Tablet**. If there is failing memory, add the **Cerebral Tonic Pills**.
- Menopausal symptoms caused by deficient Kidney Yang include symptoms of fatigue, indifference, inability to get warm, cold extremities, loose stools, frequent urination and sometimes incontinence, edema in the face or lower body and extremities, a sensation of fullness in the abdomen, failing memory, sore and weak lower back and knees, and a pale tongue with a thin coat. The best formula for this pattern is **Rehmannia Eight**.

Menstrual and Premenstrual Imbalances

Major menstrual imbalances include absent or poor menstrual flow, excessive menstrual bleeding, and painful menstruation. Premenstrual imbalances include pain, other physical symptoms, and emotional distress (irritability) that occur both before and sometimes during menstrual periods. Diagnosing menstrual or premenstrual imbalances and choosing the most appropriate herbal formulas for treatment can be very complex tasks and will often require the expertise of a trained practitioner. If you use herbal formulas on your own and don't experience some relief after several cycles, you should see a qualified practitioner to rule out the presence of any serious illness.

Menstrual Imbalances

- Absent or poor menstrual flow caused by deficient Liver and Kidneys includes symptoms of delayed menstruation past the age of eighteen or scanty menstrual flow of a pinkish color that decreases with each cycle, usually accompanied by dizziness, sore and weak lower back, ringing in the ears, a dry mouth and throat, a hot sensation in the palms and soles, night sweats, and a red tongue with little to no coat. Sometimes the individual always feels cold. The best formula choice for this pattern is **Rehmannia Six**. Where the individual always feels cold, **Rehmanna Eight** is a good choice. **Ginseng and Tang Gui Ten** may be used to enhance the effect of either of the latter formulas.

- Absent or poor menstrual flow due to deficient Qi and Blood includes symptoms of delayed menstruation or scanty menstruation that gradually stops, dizziness, pale and dull complexion, lips, and tongue, palpitations, blurred vision, poor appetite, extreme fatigue, often to the point where the individual is too tired to talk, shortness of breath, weak extremities, and loose stools. The formulas of choice are **Ginseng and Tang Gui Ten**, **Tang Gui and Ginseng Eight**, or **Ginseng and Longan**.

- Absent or poor menstrual flow due to Blood stasis and Qi stagnation includes symptoms of delayed or completely absent menstruation with depression, irritability, restlessness, a sensation of fullness in the chest and ribs, or a sensation of fullness—with pain—in the abdomen that worsens with pressure, and either a dark tongue or a tongue that has dark, raised dots. The best formulas for this imbalance is **Tang Gui Four**, possibly combined with **Bupleurum and Tang Gui**. These symptoms often presage a more serious disorder and consultation with a trained practitioner is recommended.

- Painful menstruation caused by Blood Stasis and Qi stagnation includes symptoms of lower abdominal pain or swelling before or during menstruation, scanty menstrual flow with clotted or dark blood, often accompanied by a feeling of release after large clots are expelled, painful breasts and rib areas, and a dark purplish tongue. A good formula choice is **Bupleurum and Tang Gui**, which can be combined with the **Corydalis** formula.

- Painful menstruation caused by stagnant damp and cold includes symptoms of pain in the legs, groin, and/or lower back that is relieved with heat and pressure, scanty menstrual flow with clotted or dark blood, loose stools, and a tongue with a white, greasy coat. The formula of choice is **Ginseng and Tang Gui Ten**.

- Painful menstruation caused by deficient Qi and Blood includes symptoms of a steady dull ache in the lower abdomen, during or after menstruation, that is relieved with pressure, a pale tongue and complexion, pale menstrual blood, and an attitude of indifference. The best formulas for this pattern of menstrual imbalance are **Ginseng and Longan** or **Ginseng and Tang Gui Ten**.

- Painful menstruation caused by Liver and Kidney deficiency includes symptoms of a dull pain in the lower abdomen after menstruation, a scanty, pale menstrual flow, dizziness, a sore and weak lower back, ringing in the ears, and a slightly red tongue with a thin coat. If there are more heat or deficient-Yin symptoms, use **Rehmannia Six**. If there are more cold or deficient-Yang symptoms, use **Rehmannia Eight**.

Premenstrual Imbalances

- Premenstrual imbalances caused by stagnant Liver Qi include symptoms of breast fullness and tenderness, minor abdominal swelling and pain, restlessness, irritability, and emotional sensitivity. The formula of choice is **Bupleurum and Tang Gui**.

- Premenstrual imbalances caused by deficient Spleen and Kidney Yang include symptoms of edema (fluid retention) in the face, eyelids, and extremities, possible diarrhea, abdominal fullness and pain, a sore and weak lower back and knees, an attitude of indifference, and a tongue with a white, greasy coat. The best formulas for this pattern of premenstrual imbalance are **Rehmannia Eight** and **Ginseng and Atractylodes**.

- Premenstrual imbalances caused by excess Liver fire due to deficient Blood include symptoms of headache, especially at the top of the head, dizziness, insomnia, restlessness, pains throughout the body that appear anytime around menstruation, and a red or pale tongue. The best formula choice is a combination of **Tang Gui Four** and **Bupleurum and Tang Gui**.

Obesity

Excessive weight gain is not a diagnosis in itself, but obesity tends to worsen other imbalances, such as high blood pressure, back pain, diabetes, and arteriosclerosis. In every case where weight loss is a goal, simply chewing all food completely—at least twenty to thirty chews—including soup and other liquids, will increase the metabolism of foods and reduce appetite. Oriental Medicine sees a number of causes of, and prescribes a number of treatments for, obesity.

Obesity Imbalances

- Obesity caused by excessive food intake includes symptoms of a desire to eat large quantities of food, belching, gas, a sensation of fullness in the upper abdomen, and a heavy sensation in the head. Often the body responds as if it weren't getting *enough* nutrition, because its metabolic machinery has stopped functioning properly. The best formulas for this pattern of obesity are **Citrus and Pinellia** and **Apricot Seed and Linum**.
- Obesity caused by retention of damp heat includes symptoms of a generalized heavy sensation, fullness in the chest and upper abdomen, possible edema, constipation, nausea, and dizziness. The formula of choice for this pattern is **Hoelin Five**.
- Obesity caused by Liver stagnation includes symptoms of emotional changes that lead to excessive eating and usually occur in middle age, depression, restlessness, sudden anger, headache, insomnia, a feeling of fullness in the upper abdomen and lower ribs, either loose or hard stools, but no normal stools, a bitter taste in the mouth, possible lack of appetite, and occasionally a seemingly endless thin, yellow coat on the tongue. Excellent formulas for this pattern are the **Bupleurum and Tang Gui** formula, the **Bupleurum, Inula, and Cyperus** formula, and the **Minor Bupleurum** formula.
- Obesity caused by Qi deficiency of the Spleen and Lungs includes symptoms of fatigue on mild exertion, spontaneous sweating,

shortness of breath, palpitations, loose stools, low fever or a sensation of a fever, pale complexion, and a pale and swollen tongue with a white coat. The formulas of choice are **Stephania and Astragalus** or **Major Six Herbs**.

- Obesity caused by Kidney deficiency includes symptoms of a sore and weak lower back and knees, fatigue, drowsiness, impotence or menstrual difficulties, frequent and excessive urination, and a pale and swollen tongue with a thin coat. The treatment of choice is **Rehmannia Eight**.

Perspiration

While normal perspiration isn't a problem, excessive perspiration or perspiration at the "wrong" times signals an imbalance that will eventually lead to a more serious condition.

Perspiration Imbalances

- Spontaneous perspiration caused by a disharmony of the Nourishing Qi and Protective Qi is accompanied by symptoms of an aversion to wind and drafts or to extremes of cold and hot, insomnia that worsens with strong emotional excitation, frequent colds, and a thin, white coat on the tongue. Two excellent formulas for this pattern of imbalance are **Major Four Herbs** or **Major Six Herbs**. **Panax Ginseng Capsules** may be used supplementally with either of these formulas to increase their effect of building Qi.
- Spontaneous perspiration caused by deficient Lung Qi is accompanied by symptoms of a strong aversion to cold that worsens after exertion, pale complexion, a tendency to chill easily, and frailty. The formula of choice for this pattern is **Ginseng and Astragalus**. **Panax Ginseng Capsules** may be used supplementally to increase the formula's effect of building Qi.
- Spontaneous perspiration caused by interior heat is accompanied by symptoms of strong thirst, an urge for cold drinks, a flushed complexion, fever, constipation, a feverish feeling throughout the body, sometimes with pain in the extemities, and a red tongue. The best formula for this pattern is **Rehmannia Six**.
- Night perspiration due to a deficiency of Heart Blood is accompanied by symptoms of perspiraton during sleep that stops on

awakening, insomnia, shortness of breath, palpitations, fatigue, a pale face, and a thin coat on the tongue. Two excellent formulas for this pattern are **Ginseng and Longan** and **Ginseng and Zizyphus**.

- Night perspiration due to deficient Yin fire is accompanied by symptoms of onset of fever at a specific time every day, restlessness, nervousness, insomnia, hot sensation in the palms and soles, nocturnal emissions in men and irregular menses in women, a thin body type, and a red tongue with little or no coating. A good formula for this pattern of imbalance is **Anemarrhena, Phellodendron, and Rehmannia**.

- Perspiration caused by Exhaustion is characterized by symptoms of sudden onset of excessive perspiration accompanying an acute or serious disease, exhaustion due to fighting off the disease, cold extremities, and a rigid, dry tongue. The best formulas for this pattern of imbalance are **Tang Gui and Ginseng Eight** or **Ginseng and Tang Gui Ten**. **Panax Ginseng Capsules** may be used supplementally with either formula to increase their effect of building Qi.

Trauma Caused by Surgery or Injury

Treatment for the physical trauma caused by surgery depends on the nature of the surgery itself and any attendant postsurgical therapy. This is a situation where it is best to consult first with a practitioner. If there are no postsurgical complications, and if the immune system is not being suppressed to prevent organ or tissue rejection, it is generally safe to build up the system with herbs.

- In some cases, a practitioner may want to use Blood-moving herbal formulas to speed healing. Here we suggest only herbal formulas that strengthen and tonify the body during recovery (though some may have a mild Blood-moving component). Three excellent formulas for this are **Tang Gui Four**, **Major Four Herbs**, and **Ginseng and Tang Gui Ten**. **Panax Ginseng Capsules** may be used supplementally to increase their effect of building Qi.

- If there is constipation during convalescence, the **Apricot Seed and Linum** formula may be used to increase bowel function without a strong laxative action. Care should be taken not to overuse this formula, however, because it has a mild Blood-moving effect.

- If there has been bone surgery, the **Pseudoginseng and Dragon Blood** formula may be taken to increase the speed and quality of healing of bone and tendon tissue.

For the trauma specifically caused by injury, Oriental Medicine uses a therapeutic technique called "hit medicine." In this book we include two formulas from the hit-medicine arsenal, both of which are remarkably effective.

- **Pseudoginseng and Dragon Blood** is commonly used for broken bones, muscle sprains and strains, and tendon injuries.
- **Tian Qi and Eucommia** is commonly used for back strains and injuries, knee injuries, and to strengthen the lower back.

Urinary Infections

Urinary infections are generally caused by imbalances of Qi, heat, and/or dampness. Diet is also an important contributing factor, particularly when heat is the cause of urinary infections. Where there is heat involvement, remember to avoid spicy foods, fried foods, or alcohol.

Urinary Infection Imbalances

- Pain and spasm of the urinary tract caused by heat or stones includes symptoms of painful urination with scanty flow and the sensation of an obstructed flow while urinating, a sensation of a heavy weight in the abdomen, with twitching or spasming and pain in the lower back, decreasing yellow urine, and a red tongue with a thin, yellow coat. A good formula choice for this pattern is **Dianthus**.
- Pain and spasm of the urinary tract caused by stagnant Qi includes symptoms of painful urination with scanty flow and the sensation of an obstructed flow while urinating, a sensation of fullness in the lower abdomen, and a greenish or purplish tongue. The formula of choice is **Dianthus**, to which the **Corydalis** formula may be added.
- Pain and spasm of the urinary tract due to deficient Qi includes symptoms of pain, a heaviness and a dropping feeling in the lower

abdomen, "dripping" after urination, and a pale face and tongue. A good formula choice is **Ginseng and Astragalus**, to which the **Corydalis** formula may be added.

- Pain and spasm of the urinary tract accompanied by blood in the urine is a serious condition that should be evaluated by a trained practitioner. In Oriental Medicine, this pattern is caused by damp-heat and is broken down into two distinct stages, one acute and one chronic:

  The acute stage of this damp-heat urinary tract imbalance includes symptoms of hot, burning, and painful urination with red-tinged urine and possible blood clots, sharp pain at irregular times, restlessness, and a tongue with a yellow coat. We do not recommend an herbal formula for self-treatment here, because this imbalance needs immediate evaluation by a trained practitioner.

  The chronic stage of this damp-heat urinary-tract imbalance also involves deficient Kidney Yin. Chronic damp-heat and deficient-Kidney-Yin urinary-tract infections are characterized by their recurrent nature even after repeated treatment by antibiotics. They include symptoms of dark urine with red cells on testing, a sore and weak lower back, fatigue, and a light red tongue. The best formula for this pattern is **Anemarrhena, Phellodendron, and Rehmannia**, to which **Rehmannia Six** may be added.

- Pain and spasm of the urinary tract accompanied by fat in the urine is caused by damp-heat. Again, this imbalance is broken down into two distinct stages, one acute and one chronic.

  The acute stage includes symptoms of cloudy white and scanty urine, burning and pain on urination, and a red tongue with a greasy coat. The formula of choice is **Dianthus**. If there is also prostate involvement, **Hoelen and Polyporus** is an excellent choice.

  The chronic stage of this damp-heat urinary-tract imbalance also involves deficient Kidney Yin and includes symptoms of fatty urine with less burning and pain upon urination, dizziness, fatigue, weakness and soreness in the lower back, and a small tongue. The formula of choice is **Rehmannia Six**. If there is also prostate involvement, **Hoelen and Polyporus** is the alternate choice.

- Some urinary-tract imbalances are brought on by overwork and have as their root cause acute, recurrent, and prolonged attacks of some of the imbalances outlined above that eventually lead to chronic symptoms of "dribbling" after urination, an inability to control urination, little or no urination, fatigue, and a pale tongue. Symptoms get worse with exertion and better with rest. Several formulas excellent for this pattern of urinary tract imbalance are **Ginseng and Longan**, **Ginseng and Atractylodes**, and **Stephania and Astragalus**.

Yeast Infections and Leukorrhea

In many ways, these two imbalances are viewed as one and the same since both are characterized by vaginal discharge. In Oriental Medicine, however, the term "yeast infection," and the discharge associated with it, implies that internal heat is a causal factor. Frequently, an underlying imbalance in the body leads to an overall weakness that allows yeast to proliferate. The long-term effect of such yeast proliferation is chronic and stagnant damp-heat conditions.

The discharge of leukorrhea, on the other hand, is often not heat-related and may even be considered normal. When the discharge is excessive and accompanied by a bad odor, or if there is itching or burning, then leukorrhea is viewed as a deficiency-related imbalance.

The guidelines below will help you distinguish between the two imbalances and choose the proper formula.

Yeast Infection and Leukorrhea Imbalances

- Yeast infections caused by damp-heat conditions include symptoms of profuse yellow and foul-smelling vaginal discharge that is sticky, fetid, or bloody and has a muddy quality, itching, lower abdominal pain, scanty urination, a strong thirst, a dry, bitter taste in the mouth, and a red tongue with a yellow coat. A good formula for this pattern of imbalance is **Gentiana**.
- Leukorrhea caused by Spleen deficiency and Liver stagnation includes symptoms of profuse white or light yellowish vaginal discharge that has no odor and is sticky to the touch, a pale complexion, cold extremities, poor appetite, loose stools, possible depression, and a pale tongue with a white, greasy-looking coat. The best formula for this pattern of imbalance is **Ginseng and Atractylodes**.

- Leukorrhea caused by Kidney deficiency includes symptoms of profuse and watery white vaginal discharge, sore and weak lower back, a cold sensation in the lower abdominal area, clear urination that is more frequent at night, loose stools, and a pale tongue with a thin, white coat. The formulas of choice for this pattern of imbalance are **Rehmannia Eight** or **Tang Gui and Ginseng Eight**.

Note: The **Tang Gui and Indigo** formula has been found very useful in treating leukorrhea when combined with any of the other suggested formulas.

Appendix A

Glossary of Oriental Medicine Terms

Acupressure: Chinese healing treatment that uses hand and finger pressure and massage on meridian points and channels on the skin to stimulate energy in the body and provide symptomatic relief. Acupressure is similar to acupuncture, but employs no needles, and thus it is more limited in scope and effectiveness.

Acupuncture: Chinese healing treatment that uses thin sterile needles inserted into specific meridian points on the skin to stimulate energy in the body, encourage homeostatis of hormone function and Organ interaction, and give symptomatic relief of pain.

Acupuncture Points: Specific locations along the skin where Qi meridians (channels) run closest to the surface of the body. These points are stimulated by needles or touch to facilitate the circulation of Qi and Blood, encourage proper Organ function, relieve pain, encourage homeostatis of hormone function and Organ interaction, and give symptomatic relief of pain.

Affinity: One of the four healing properties of herbs. Every herb has a specific affinity for one or more Yin or Yang Organs.

Air Qi: The Qi received from the air we breathe.

Astringe: An herb's therapeutic ability to consolidate, concentrate, hold, or condense weak and deficient Qi, Blood, Essence (Jing), Spirit (Shen), and/or Fluids. Also to dry up excess Damp imbalances. Herbs that astringe help the body retain essential fluids and energies, and strengthen tissues and Organs. In the simplest terms, such herbs "plug up" any "holes" in the body from which energy is leaking.

Balance (Harmony): In Oriental Medicine, the state of good health—also called harmony—which results from the vibrant and harmonious interaction of Yin and Yang energies.

Blood: One of the five essential energies of the body in Oriental Medicine. Blood is the physical manifestation of Qi and is responsible for carrying nourishment and moisture to the Organs, tissues, and muscles.

Channels: Also called "meridians," these are nonmaterial pathways that run along the surface of the body and are connected via Qi energy to specific Organs. The channels are utilized for treatment both in herbal medicine and in acupuncture.

Climates: In Oriental Medicine, the name given to the primary external causes of illness or imbalance, which include Wind, Heat, Cold, Dryness, Dampness, and Summer Heat or Fire. The latter are also called the Six Evils. External causes of illness can progress and penetrate to the interior of the body, where they then become internal wind, internal heat, internal cold, internal damp, etc.

Cold: An external or internal "climatic" imbalance or ailment characterized by chills, aversion to cold, lethargy and fatigue, loose stools or diarrhea, and profuse, clear urination. Cold can also penetrate to the interior of the body, resulting in internal-cold conditions. Cold is yin in character.

Damp: An external or internal "climatic" imbalance or ailment characterized by fluid accumulations, swelling and distension, particularly of abdomen, diarrhea, a feeling of heaviness in chest, heavy expectoration and discharges, and joint pains. Damp can also penetrate to the interior of the body, and often combines with heat and cold, resulting in internal damp-heat or damp-cold conditions. A condition of dampness often indicates a breakdown in a fundamental metabolic process within the body: fluids simply do not act the way they are supposed to. An apt metaphor might be a broken iron that instead of steam produces only dripping water.

Decoction: *(tang)* In Oriental Medicine, the method of boiling down herbs to create a simple broth or tea that may be taken medicinally.

Deficiency: Insufficient quantities of and/or weak functioning of Qi, Blood, Essence (Jing), Spirit (Shen), Fluids and/or Organs resulting in imbalance and illness. For example, deficient Blood does not adequately nourish organs, tissues, and muscles. Deficient Qi prevents Blood, Fluids, and Organs from performing their proper tasks.

Diagnosis: In Oriental Medicine, the method of diagnosing illness through the process of listening, smelling, interviewing, and touching the patient, and observing how they look, dress, and act.

Dispel: An herb's therapeutic ability to disperse, move, circulate, and/or redistribute stagnant Qi, Blood, Fluids, and phlegm, or imbalances of Wind, Heat, Cold, Damp, and Fire that are present externally or internally.

Effect: One of the four healing properties of herbs. Every herb has a specific effect or action in the body. Herbs either dispel, astringe, purge, or tonify Qi, Blood, Fluids, phlegm, and external or internal causes of illness or imbalance.

Eight Principles of Diagnosis: Oriental Medicine's eight-prong system of diagnosing illnesses by their yin or yang, cold or hot, deficient or excess, and internal or external natures. (See separate entries for each of eight conditions.)

Empty Heat: Also called "False Heat." A condition of internal heat in the body that is caused by a deficiency of Yin. Empty heat symptoms include diarrhea and cold extremities (yin conditions), but there is usually a fever with flushed or red face (yang conditions) and no aversion to the cold. Despite the presence of fever, warming herbs are usually required to treat the overall yin deficiency.

Energy: A broad term used in Oriental Medicine and other alternative health disciplines to describe both the nonmaterial and material vital forces that both create and sustain the life of the body. In Oriental Medicine, Qi is pure energy and is also the driving and fundamental life force within the individual. Blood is another vital energy of the body, but it also has a physical aspect.

Essence: (Jing) The primordial energy all individuals are born with, similar to DNA, and responsible for the fundamental growth and reproductive processes of the body. One of the five basic energy substances of the body.

Excess: Overfunction (hyperactivity) of Organs and/or Organ systems in the body possibly due to stagnation of Qi, Blood, Essence (Jing), Spirit (Shen), and/or Fluids, resulting in imbalances or illness in the body; hyperfunction of any of the Organs and/or Organ systems.

Exterior: In Oriental Medicine's diagnostic system, exterior symptoms of an illness or imbalance occur either on the surface of the body—in skin, hair, or nails—or in tissues, muscles, joints, nerves, blood vessels, or Organ systems near the surface of, as opposed to deep within, the body.

External (Disharmony/Imbalance): Refers to the external causes of an illness (disharmony or imbalance): Wind, Heat, Cold, Dryness, Dampness, Summer Heat or Fire. (See "Climates.")

False Heat: A condition of internal heat caused by a yin deficiency. See "Empty Heat."

Fire: An extreme condition of internal heat, often accompanied by severe emotional excesses, called "inner-fire symptoms," such as extreme anger or rage. May also be brought on by overindulgence in certain foods and alcohol. Symptoms include severe dehydration, skin rashes, red eyes and face, sparse urine, constipation, mental agitation and/or delirium. Fire especially affects Lungs, Liver, and Stomach.

Five Elements System: A complex system that organizes all the processes in nature, and the interaction between living organisms and nature, into five categories called Wind, Fire, Earth, Metal, and Water. Illness is also classified according to these five categories. In this book, we use the Eight Principles of diagnosis as our focal point, and not the Five Elements (also called the Five

Phases). Many of the books in the bibliography contain excellent discussions of the Five Elements System.

Flavor: See "Taste," one of the four healing properties of herbs.

Fluids (Jin Ye): Also called "Moisture." Jin fluids are lighter fluids that moisten the Lungs, skin, and muscles and that work with Protective Qi to help protect the surface of the body. Ye fluids are heavier fluids that work with the Kidneys and Spleen to help Nourishing Qi. Fluids may become deficient (e.g., in conditions of dehydration and constipation), or they may accumulate (e.g., in conditions of congestion and edema). Phlegm or mucus is also a condition of accumulated fluids. See "Phlegm."

Food Qi: The Qi received from the foods and liquids we ingest.

Harmony: Also called "balance." Refers to the state of good health resulting from the harmonious interaction of yin and yang that produces strong, healthy Qi.

Heat: An external or internal "climatic" imbalance or ailment characterized by fever, aversion to heat, overactivity, constipation, dehydration, sparse dark urination, and insomnia. Heat can also progress and penetrate to the interior of the body and frequently combines with damp to create internal heat-damp imbalances. Heat is Yang in character.

Herbal Properties: An herb is therapeutically categorized by its four healing properties: nature, taste, affinity with specific organs, and effect or action in the body.

Imbalance: The term used in Oriental Medicine to characterize illness, resulting from a fundamental imbalance between yin and yang energies that results in secondary imbalances in Qi, Blood, Essence (Jing), Spirit (Shen), Fluids, and/or Organs.

Interior: According to Oriental Medicine's diagnostic system, interior symptoms of illness or imbalance occur in Organs, Organ systems, major blood vessels, and other organic systems found deep within the body, as opposed to on or near the surface. (See "Exterior.")

Internal: (Disharmony/Imbalance) Refers to the seven primary internal or emotional causes of illness or imbalance: Anger, Sadness, Grief, Fear, Fright, Joy, and Rumination.

Jing: Chinese term for "Essence," one of the five basic energies of the body. (See "Essence.")

Jin Ye: See "Fluids."

Materia Medica: Any large compendium of Chinese herbs—plant, animal, or mineral in origin—that categorizes them by their botanical and/or biological characteristics and by their healing properties.

Meridian: Nonmaterial pathways, also called channels, that run along the surface of the body and are connected via Qi energy to specific Organs. The meridians organize the body's functions and are utilized for diagnosis and treatment both in herbal medicine and in acupuncture.

Moisture: The essential Jin Ye Fluids of the body. (See "Fluids.")

Mucus: See "Phlegm."

Nature: One of the four active healing properties of herbs. Herbs possess three essential natures: warm or hot (yang); cool or cold (yin); and neutral.

Nutritive Qi: The Qi energy that provides nourishment to the Organs and tissues of the body.

Organs: In Oriental Medicine, there are twelve major Organs in the body, six of which are yin and six of which are yang in nature. (See "Yin Organs" and "Yang Organs.") In this book, we capitalize Organ names to emphasize the fact that in Oriental Medicine, they are important not only for their anatomical properties, but because they embody complex energy systems that are crucial to many functions within the body.

Organ Qi: The Qi energy unique to each Organ and Organ function. In illness or imbalance, Organ Qi may be deficient, stagnant, sinking, or rebellious, depending on the specific yin/yang imbalance.

Original Qi: The prenatal Qi with which we are born, mostly received from our parents via heredity and during pregnancy.

Palpation: Light massage and/or stronger finger-and-hand pressure performed by traditional practitioner on the skin and other parts of the body along meridian points and channels that correspond to specific Organs. Palpation allows the practitioner to make a general assessment of body temperature and skin condition, determine where there may be areas of poor muscle tone and/or pain, and diagnose possible Organ disharmonies.

Phlegm: Phlegm or "mucus" is a condition of accumulated Fluids that may have either a material aspect (e.g., chest, Lung, and sinus congestion, many kinds of tumors, and plaque deposits in the circulatory system), or a nonmaterial aspect (e.g., high blood pressure).

Protective Qi: The Qi that circulates on the outside of the body to protect it from illnesses and imbalances caused by external or climatic conditions. Also called "Surface Qi."

Pulse Taking: The more than two-thousand-year-old science of sphygmology, a diagnostic system used to detect an individual's past and present imbalances and illnesses by reading twelve major wrist pulses, each of which corresponds to one of the twelve major Organs.

Purge: An herb's therapeutic ability to eliminate, expel, and/or detoxify where there is obstruction, chronic stagnation, or "poison" (toxicity) in Qi, Blood, Fluids, and phlegm, or where there are external or internal balances of especially Heat, Damp, and Fire.

Qi: The fundamental life force or energy that is found in all living things and is formed from the interaction of yin and yang energies.

Qigong: A five-thousand-year-old Chinese system of physical movements and controlled breathing designed to consolidate and promote the free flow of Qi energy throughout the body both to enhance physical well-being and activate self-healing.

Rebellious Qi: Qi that flows in the wrong direction. (Gastric reflux is an example of Rebellious Qi.)

San Jiao: See "Triple Warmer."

Shen: Chinese term for "Spirit" or "Mind." (See "Spirit.")

Spirit (Shen): The higher consciousness involved in creative and mental activities. Sometimes called "Soul," Spirit is one of the five basic energy substances of the body and may be either strong (calm) or weak (agitated).

Stagnant Qi: Qi that is "stuck" and doesn't flow freely. Occurs when the normal flow of Qi either slows down or is blocked by deficiency (not enough flow), excess (too much flow), or injury (obstruction to flow).

T'ai Chi Chuan: Chinese system of martial arts consisting of a series of slow-movement physical exercises designed to concentrate and promote the flow of Qi and Blood.

Tao: The Chinese system of philosophy and religion that views everything in the universe as interrelated and striving toward harmonious balance, with no beginning and no end. Within this system, individuals are microcosms of the universe, subject to the same interactive energies that move toward harmony and balance.

Taste: One of the four healing properties of herbs. Herbs possess five distinct tastes, each of which has a specific healing character: sour, bitter, sweet or bland, spicy, and salty.

Three Treasures: In Oriental Medicine, the collective term used to describe Qi, Essence (Jing), and Spirit (Shen). When Qi, Essence, and Spirit are vital, healthy, and harmonious, a person is said to enjoy perfect health.

Tonify: An herb's therapeutic ability to nourish, harmonize, support, and invigorate stagnant and deficient conditions of Qi, Blood, Essence (Jing), Spirit (Shen), Fluids, and Organs.

Triple Warmer: Also called "Triple Burner" and *San Jiao* in Chinese. In Oriental Medicine, this is a yang organ or, more precisely, an "energy system," that has no equivalent in conventional medicine. The Triple Warmer is crucial to all phases of digestion and has three parts: the Upper Burner (from mouth to Stomach); the Middle Burner (from stomach to Large Intestine); and the Lower Burner (from Small Intestine to rectum).

Wind: Wind is one of the major external and internal causes of illness or imbalance and is characterized by symptoms of shaking, trembling, dizziness, and joint and muscle pains that move throughout the body. Wind symptoms are sudden and acute, frequently occur in the spring, and commonly occur in tandem with other external causes of illness, especially cold.

Yang: One of the two fundamental polar energies found in all living things. Yang qualities or conditions are hot, dry, excessive, and on or near the surface of the body. Yang complements yin.

Yang Organs: The six hollow yang organs include the Large Intestine, Small Intestine, Bladder, Gallbladder, Stomach, and Triple Warmer. These organs are found closer to the surface of the body and are all gastrointestinal in function.

Yin: One of the two fundamental polar energies found in all living things. Yin qualities or conditions are cold, damp, deficient, and found in the interior of the body. Yin complements yang.

Yin Organs: The six solid yin organs include the Lungs, Heart, Liver, Kidneys, Spleen, and Pericardium. These organs are considered the most important in Oriental Medicine. They are found deep within the body and are responsible for manufacturing, storing, and regulating Qi, Blood, Essence (Jing), Spirit (Shen), and Fluids.

Yin-Yang: In Chinese theory, the fundamental principle of two mutually interdependent and constantly interacting polar energies that sustain all living organisms. The interaction of Yin and Yang produces Qi.

Zangfu Organs: *Zangfu* is the Chinese term used in Oriental Medicine to characterize the body's complete Organ system. The *Zangfu* include the six solid yin organs (*Zang*), which are located deep within the body and are responsible for manufacturing, storing, and regulating Qi, Blood, Essence (Jing), Spirit (Shen), and Fluids; and the six hollow yang organs (*Fu*), which are found closer to the surface of the body and which are all gastrointestinal in function.

Appendix B

Herb Suppliers

The raw herbs and herbal formulas in this book are readily available in many of the herb shops found in Chinatowns in major cities in the United States. However, if you don't live near one of these cities, or don't wish to travel farther than your phone to purchase herbs, the following suppliers will ship them to you.

This is a short list for several reasons. Few herbal suppliers have the staff necessary to fulfill individual orders, and many don't like dealing directly with the public, particularly if the buyer is not a licensed practitioner or there are language barriers. Most suppliers deal directly with practitioners who order herbs in large lots for their practices, have experience dealing with Chinese-speaking suppliers, and can order herbs in both Chinese and Latin.

Both the suppliers below, however, provide excellent service, are fluent in English, and can deliver herbs quickly (overnight or second-day delivery).

Tian Ming Herbs
P.O. Box 244
Whitehall, PA 18015-0244
(888) 219-2221 (toll-free) or (610) 266-6110
Fax: (610) 266-5156

Provides ready-made herbal formulas in pill and powder form. They will take orders directly over the phone, or they will mail or fax you an order form. Visa and MasterCard are accepted.

China Herbs
6333 Wayne Avenue
Philadelphia, PA 19144
(800) 221-4372 (toll-free) or (215) 843-5864
Fax: (215) 849-3338

Provides raw herbs—separated, weighed, packaged, and labeled—so you can prepare herbal formulas at home. Also carry ready-made preparations in powder form. They will take orders directly over the phone, or they will mail or fax you an order form. Visa and MasterCard are accepted.

Occasionally there are delays getting certain herbs since they are shipped from overseas. However, both suppliers will go out of their way to make sure you get the herbs and formulas you want when you need them.

Appendix C

Information Resources

For referrals to qualified Oriental Medicine practitioners and acupuncturists, please call the **American Association of Oriental Medicine (AAOM)** at (610) 266-1433, or fax them at (610) 264-2768. They may also be reached via E-mail at AAOM1@aol.com.

Additional referrals and other information about Oriental Medicine can be found at the AAOM World Wide Web site. The address is http://www.aaom.org.

The AAOM also distributes several publications, including an updated listing of schools of acupuncture and Oriental Medicine in the United States and Canada, and the newly published "Naeser Laser Carpal Tunnel Booklet," a guide to home treatment of carpal tunnel syndrome using acupuncture points.

Other information resources for Oriental Medicine and Chinese herbal medicine include:

Accrediting Commission for Acupuncture and Oriental Medicine
1010 Wayne Avenue, Suite 1270
Silver Spring, MD 20910
Phone: (301) 608-9680
Fax: (301) 608-9576

American Foundation of Traditional Chinese Medicine
505 Beach Street
San Francisco, CA 94133
(415) 776-0502

American Journal of Acupuncture
P.O. Box 610
Capitola, CA 95010
Phone/Fax: (408) 475-1439

Council of Colleges of Acupuncture and Oriental Medicine
1010 Wayne Avenue, Suite 1270
Silver Spring, MD 20910
Phone: (301) 608-9175

Institute for Traditional Medicine
2017 SE Hawthorne Boulevard
Portland, OR 97214
http://www.europa.com/~itm

Journal of Chinese Medicine
c/o Eastland Press
1260 Activity Drive, #A
Vista, CA 92083
Phone: (800) 453-3278

Journal of Oriental Medicine in America
16161 Ventura Boulevard, Suite 406
Encino, CA 91436
Phone: (888) 556-5662
Fax: (818) 345-9035 (local only)

National Certification Commission of Acupuncture and Oriental Medicine
P.O. Box 97075
Washington, DC 20090-7075
Phone: (202) 232-1404
Fax: (202) 462-6157

Oriental Healing Arts Institute
1945 Palo Verde Avenue, Suite 208
Long Beach, CA 90815

Oriental Medicine Magazine
3723 N. Southport
Chicago, IL 60613
Phone: (312) 871-0342
Fax: (312) 248-7427

Protocol Journal of Botanical Medicine
P.O. Box 108
Harvard, MA 01451
Phone: (800) 466-5422

Appendix D

Selected Bibliography

Beinfield, Harriet and Efrem Korngold. *Between Heaven and Earth: A Guide to Chinese Medicine*. New York: Ballantine Books, 1991.

Bensky, Dan and Andrew Gamble, with Ted Kaptchuk. *Chinese Herbal Medicine Materia Medica*. Seattle: Eastland Press, 1986; 1993.

Bensky, Dan and Randall Barolet. *Chinese Herbal Medicine: Formulas and Strategies*. Seattle: Eastland Press, 1990.

Chun-han Zhu. *Clinical Handbook of Chinese Prepared Medicine*. Brookline, MA: Paradigm Publications, 1989.

Dharmananda, Subhuti. *Pearls from the Golden Cabinet: The Practitioner's Guide to the Use of Chinese Herbs and Traditional Formulas*. Long Beach, CA: Oriental Healing Arts Institute, 1988.

Dharmananda, Subhuti. *Chinese Herbology: A Professional Training Program*. Portland, OR: Institute for Traditional Medicine, 2016 S.E. Hawthorne, Portland, OR 97214, 1994.

Ehling, Dagmar, with Steve Smart. *The Chinese Herbalist's Handbook*. Santa Fe: Inwood Press, 1994.

Fan, Warner J. W. *A Manual of Chinese Herbal Medicine: Principles and Practice for Easy Reference*. Boston: Shambhala, 1996.

Fratkin, Jake. *Chinese Herbal Patent Formulas : A Practical Guide*. Santa Fe: Shya Publications, 1986.

Hadady, Letha. *The Asian Way to Wellness: Your Personal Guide to Using Asian Herbal Treatments for Daily Well-Being.* New York: Crown Publishers, 1996.

Him-che Yeung. *Handbook of Chinese Herbs and Formulas.* Los Angeles: 1983.

———. *Handbook Of Chinese Herbs.* Rosemead: Institute of Chinese Medicine, 1996.

Hong-yen Hsu. *Oriental Materia Medica: A Concise Guide.* Long Beach, CA: Oriental Healing Arts Institute, 1986.

———. *How to Treat Yourself with Chinese Herbs.* New Canaan, CT: Keats Publishing and Oriental Healing Arts Institute, 1993.

Hong-yen Hsu and Chau-shin Hsu. *Commonly Used Chinese Herb Formulas with Illustrations.* Long Beach, CA: Oriental Healing Arts Institute, 1990.

Huang, Kee Chang. *The Pharmacology of Chinese Herbs.* Boca Raton, FL: CRC Press, 1993.

Hyatt, Richard. *Chinese Herbal Medicine: Ancient Art and Modern Science.* New York, NY: Schocken Books, 1978.

Kun-Ying Yen, *The Illustrated Chinese Materia Medica: Crude and Prepared.* Taipei: SMC Publishing Inc., 1992.

Le, Kim. *The Simple Path to Health: A Guide to Oriental Nutrition and Well-Being.* Portland, OR: Rudra Press, 1996.

McNamara, Sheila. *Traditional Chinese Medicine.* New York, NY: Basic Books, 1996.

Mowrey, Daniel B. *Next Generation Herbal Medicine.* New Canaan, CT: Keats Publishing, 1990.

———. *The Scientific Validation of Herbal Medicine.* New Canaan, CT: Keats Publishing and Cormorant Books, 1986.

Naeser, Margaret A. *Outline Guide to Chinese Herbal Patent Medicines in Pill Form.* Boston, MA: Boston Chinese Medicine, 1990.

Reid, Daniel. *A Handbook of Chinese Healing Herbs.* Boston, MA: Shambhala, 1995.

———. *Chinese Herbal Medicine.* Boston, MA: Shambhala: 1993.

Teeguarden, Ron. *Chinese Tonic Herbs.* Tokyo: Japan Publications, 1985.

Williams, Tom. *The Complete Illustrated Guide to Chinese Medicine.* Rockport, MA: Element Books, 1996.

Yang, Kris K. and Diana X. H. Deng. *Symptoms and Treatments by Using Traditional Chinese Herbal Formulas.* Taichung: Min Tong Medicine Journal, 1996.

Appendix E

Listing of Single Herbs

No.	Common English or Latin Name	Latin Plant Name	Pinyin Mandarin Name
1	Achyranthes	Achyranthes Bidentata	Niu Xi
2	Aconite	Aconitum Carmichaeli Preparata	Fu Zi
3	Acorus	Acori Graminei	Chang Pu or Shi Chang Pu
4	Agastache	Agastache seu Pogostemi	Huo Xiang
5	Akebia	Akebia Caulis	Mu Tong
6	Albizza	Albizza Julibrissin	He Huan Pi
7	Alismatis	Alismatis Plantago-Aquaticae	Ze Xie
8	Alpina	Alpiniae Oxyphyllae	Yi Zhi Ren
9	Amber	Succinum	Hu Po
10	Anemarrhena	Anemarrhenae Asphodeloidis	Zhi Mu
11	Angelica Du Huo	Angelica Pubescens	Du Huo
12	Angelica Dahurica	Angelica Dahurica	Bai Zhi
13	Angelica Sinensis	Angelica Sinensis	Tang Gui
14	Antelope Horn	Cornu Antelopis	Ling Yang Jiao
15	Apricot Seed	Pruni Armeniacae	Xing Ren or Ku Xing Ren

No.	Common English or Latin Name	Latin Plant Name	Pinyin Mandarin Name
16	Aquilaria	Aquilariae Agallocha	Chen Xiang
17	Areca Husk	Arecae Catechu	Da Fu Pi
18	Arisaema	Arisaema Amurense	Tain Nan Xing
19	Asarum	Asarum Sieboldi	Xi Xin
20	Asparagus	Asparagi Cochinchinensis	Tian Men Dong
21	Astragalus	Astragali	Huang Qi
22	Atractylodes	Atractylodes Lancea	Cang Zhu
23	Atractylodes Alba	Atractylodes Macrocephalae	Bai Zhu
24	Auranti Fructus	Aurantii or Citri seu Ponciri	Zhi Ke
25	Auranti Immaturus	Aurantii Immaturus	Zhi Shi
26	Avicularis	Polygoni Avicularis	Bian Xu
27	Bamboo Leaf	Lophatheri Gracilis	Dan Zhu Ye
28	Biota	Biota Orientalis	Bai Zi Ren
29	Bupleurum	Bupleuri Radix	Chai Hu
30	Burdock Fructus	Arctii Lappae	Niu Bang Zi
31	Capillaris	Artemesia Capillaris	Yin Chen Hao
32	Cardamom Seed (ripe)	Amomi Fructus seu Semen	Sha Ren
33	Cardamom Seed (immature)	Amomi Cardamomi	Bai Dou Kou
34	Carthamus Flower	Carthami Tinctorii	Hong Hua
35	Chrysanthemum	Chrysanthemi Morifolii	Ju Hua
36	Chrysanthemum (wild)	Chrysanthemi Indici	Ye Ju Hua
37	Cimicifuga	Cimicifugae	Sheng Ma
38	Cinnamon Bark	Cinnamomi Cassiae	Rou Gui
39	Cinnamon Twig	Cinnamomi Cassiae	Gui Zhi
40	Cistanches	Cistanches	Rou Cong Rong
41	Citri Immaturi	Citri Reticulatae Viride	Qing Pi
42	Citron, Finger Fructus	Fructus Citri Sarcodactylis	Fou Shou
43	Citrus Peel (aged)	Citri Reticulatae	Chen Pi
44	Codonopsis	Codonopsis Pilosulae	Dang Shen
45	Coix	Coicis Lachryma-Jobi	Yi Yi Ren
46	Coptis	Coptidis	Huang Lian
47	Cornu Cervi	Cornu Cervi Parvum	Lu Rong
48	Cornus	Corni Officinalis	Shan Zhu Yu
49	Corydalis	Corydalis Ambigua	Yan Hu Suo
50	Curcuma	Curcumae	Jiang Huang
51	Cuscuta	Cuscutae	Tu Si Zi
52	Cyperus	Cyperi Rotundi	Xiang Fu

No.	Common English or Latin Name	Latin Plant Name	Pinyin Mandarin Name
53	Dianthus	Dianthi	Qu Mai
54	Dioscoria	Dioscoria Oppositae	Shan Yao
55	Dipsacus	Dipsaci	Xu Duan
56	Dolichos	Dolichoris Lablab	Bian Dou or Bai Bian Dou
57	Dragon Blood	Sanguis Draconis	Xue Jie
58	Dragon Bone	Os Draconis	Long Gu
59	Dragon Teeth	Dens Draconis	Long Chi
60	Eclipta	Ecliptae Prostratae	Han Lian Cao
61	Ephedra	Ephedra Sinensis	Ma Huang
62	Eucommia Bark	Eucommiae Ulmoidis	Du Zhong
63	Evodia	Evodia Rutaecarpae	Wu Zhu Yu
64	Fennel	Foeniculi Vulgaris	Xiao Hui Xiang or Hui Xiang
65	Forsythia Fruit	Forsythia Suspensae	Lian Qiao
66	Frankincense Gum	Gummi Olibanum	Ru Xiang
67	Fritillaria	Fritillariae Cirrhosae	Chuan Bei Mu
68	Gardenia Fruit	Gardenia Jasminoidis	Zhi Zi
69	Gastrodia	Gastrodia Elatae	Tian Ma
70	Gelatinum Asini	Gelatinum Asini	E Jiao
71	Gentiana Macro	Gentiana Macrophyllae	Qin Jiao
72	Gentiana Scabra	Gentianae Scabrae	Long Dan Cao
73	Ginger (fresh)	Zingiberis Officinalis	Sheng Jiang
74	Gingko Biloba	Gingko Biloba	Ying Xing
75	Ginseng	Panax Ginseng	Ren Shen
76	Grifola	Polypori Umbellati	Zhu Ling
77	Haliotidis	Concha Haliotidis	Shi Kue Ming
78	Inula	Inula	Xuan Fu Hua
79	Isatidis	Isatidis seu Baphicacanthi	Ban Lan Gen
80	Juncus	Junci Effusi	Deng Xin Cao
81	Leonaris	Leonuri Heterophylli	Yi Mu Cao
82	Licorice	Glycyrrhizae Uralensis	Gan Cao
83	Ligusticum	Ligustici Wallichii	Chuan Xiong
84	Ligustrum	Ligustri Lucidi	Nu Zhen Zi
85	Linum	Cannabis Sativae	Huo Ma Ren
86	Longan (Arillis)	Arillis Euphoriae Longanae	Long Yan Rou
87	Lonicera Flower	Lonicerae Japonicae	Jin Yin Hua
88	Loranthus	Loranthi seu Visci	Sang Ji Sheng
89	Lotus Seed	Nelumbinis	Lian Zi
90	Lumbricus	Lumbricus	Di Long

No.	Common English or Latin Name	Latin Plant Name	Pinyin Mandarin Name
91	Lycium	Lycii Chinensis	Gou Qi Zi
92	Lysimachia (Desmodium)	Glechoma Longituba	Jin Qian Cao
93	Magnetitum	Magnetitum	Ci Shi
94	Magnolia Bark	Magnoliae Officinalis	Hou Po
95	Magnolia Flower	Magnolia Liliflorae	Xin Yi Hua
96	Marguerite Concha	Margaritaferae, Concha	Zhen Zhu Mu
97	Massa Fermenta (preparation)	Massa Fermentata	Shenqu
98	Moutan	Moutan Radicis	Mu Dan Pi
99	Myrrh Gum	Myrrha	Mo Yao
100	Nelumbinus Stamen	Nelumbinus	Lian Xu
101	Notoptergi	Notopterygii	Qiang-Huo or Chiang-Huo
102	Ophiopogon	Ophiopogonis Japonici	Mai Men Dong
103	Oyster Shell	Concha Ostreae	Mu Li
104	Peony Alba	Paeoniae Lactiflorae	Bai Shao
105	Peony Rubra	Paeoniae Rubra	Chi Shao
106	Peppermint	Mentha Arvensis	Bo He
107	Perilla Leaf	Perillae Frutescentis	Zi Su Ye
108	Phellodendron	Phellodendri	Huang Bai
109	Pinellia	Pinelliae Ternatae	Ban Xia
110	Plantago Seed	Plantaginis	Che Qian Zi
111	Platycodon	Platycodi Grandiflori	Jie Geng
112	Polygala	Polygalae Tenuifoliae	Yuan Zi
113	Polygonum Multiflorum	Polygoni Multiflori	He Shou Wu
114	Poria	Poria Cocos	Fu Ling
115	Prunella	Prunellae Vulgaris	Xia Ku Cao
116	Pseudoginseng	Pseudoginseng	San Qi, or Tian Qi
117	Pueraria	Puerariae	Ge Gen
118	Rehmannia (raw)	Rehmanniae Glutinosae	Sheng Di Huang
119	Rehmannia (steamed)	Rehmanniae Glutinosae Conquitae	Shu Di Huang
120	Rhubarb	Rheum Palmatum	Da Huang
121	Salvia	Salviae Miltiorrhizae	Dan Shen
122	Sandalwood	Santali Albi	Tan Xiang
123	Saussurea	Saussureae seu Vladimiriae	Mu Xiang
124	Schisandra	Schizandrae Chinensis	Wu Wei Zi
125	Schizonepeta	Schizonepetae Tenufoliae	Jing Jie

No.	Common English or Latin Name	Latin Plant Name	Pinyin Mandarin Name
126	Scirpus	Sparganii	San Leng
127	Scrophularia	Scrophulariae Ningpoensis	Xuan Shen
128	Scutellaria	Scutellariae Baiclaensis	Huang Qin
129	Siler	Ledebouriellae Sesloidis	Fang Feng
130	Soja Seed	Sojae Praeparatum	Dan Dou Chi
131	Sophora	Sophora Japonicae Immaturus	Huai Hua Mi
132	Stephania	Stephania Tetrandrae	Han Fang Ji
133	Talc	Talcum	Hua Shi
134	Tribuli	Tribuli Terrestris	Bai Ji Li or Ci Ji Li or Ji Li
135	Uncaria	Uncariae Cum Uncis	Gou Teng
136	Walnut	Juglandis Regiae	Hu Tao Ren
137	Xanthium	Xanthii	Can Er Zi
138	Ziziphi Fruit	Ziziphi Jujubae	Da Zao
139	Ziziphi Seed	Ziziphi Spinosae	Suan Zao Ren

Appendix F

Listing of Herbal Formulas

No.	Common English (Latin/Chinese) Name	Pinyin Mandarin Name
1	Agastache Formula	Huo Shang Zheng Qi Wan
2	Anemarrhena, Phellodendron, and Rehmannia Formula	Zhi Bai Di Huang Wan
3	Angelica Formula	Tang Gui Pian
4	Apricot and Fritillaria Formula	San She Dan Chuan Bei Ye
5	Apricot Seed and Linum Formula	Ma Zi Ren Wan
6	Bupleurum and Dragon Bone Formula	Chai Hu Jia Long Gu Mu Li Tang
7	Bupleurum, Inula, and Cyperus Formula	Shu Gan Wan
8	Bupleurum and Tang Gui Formula	Xiao Yao Wan
9	Cerebral Tonic Pills	Bu Nao Wan
10	Cimicafuga Formula	Yi Zi Tang
11	Citrus and Pinellia Formula	Er Chen Wan
12	Clematis and Stephania Formula	Shu Jing Huo Xue Tang
13	Cnidium and Tea Formula	Chuan Qiong Cha Tiao Wan
14	Concha Marguerita and Ligustrum Formula	An Shen Bu Xin Wan
15	Corydalis Formula	Shao Yao Gan Cao Tang and Yan Hu Suo

No.	Common English (Latin/Chinese) Name	Pinyin Mandarin Name
16	Corydalis Tuber Formula	Yan Hu Suo Zhi Tong Pian
17	Cyperus and Ligusticum Formula	Yue Ju Wan
18	Dianthus Formula	Ba Zheng San
19	Eight Immortal Long Life Pill	Ba Xian Chang Shou Wan
20	Fritillaria Extract Tablet	Chuan Bei Jing Pian
21	Gentiana Formula	Long Dan Xie Gan Wan
22	Ginseng and Astragalus Formula	Bu Zhong Yi Qi Wan
23	Ginseng and Atractylodes Formula	Shen Ling Bai Zhu Pian
24	Ginseng and Longan Formula	Gui Pi Tang
25	Ginseng and Tang Gui Ten Formula	Shi Quan Da Bu Wan
26	Ginseng and Zizyphus Formula	Tian Wang Bu Xin Wan
27	Hoelen and Polyporus Formula	Zhi Zhuo Gu Ben Wan
28	Hoelin Five Formula	Wu Lin San
29	Ilex and Evodia Formula	Ganmaoling
30	Leonuris and Achyranthes Formula	Jiang Ya Wan (Hypertension Pills)
31	Lonicera and Forsythia Formula	Yin Chiao Chieh Tu Pien
32	Ma Huang Formula	Ma Huang Tang
33	Major Four Herbs Formula	Si Jun Zi Tang
34	Major Six Herbs Formula	Liu Jun Zi Tang
35	Minor Bupleurum Formula	Xiao Chai Hu Tang
36	Panax Ginseng Capsules	Renshen Wan
37	Peony and Licorice Formula	Shao Yao Gan Cao Tang
38	Polygonum Tablet	He Shou Wu Pian
39	Prunella and Scutellaria Formula	Jian Ya Ping Pian
40	Pseudoginseng and Dragon Blood Formula	Chin Koo Tieh Shang Wan
41	Pueraria Combination	Ge Gen Tang
42	Qiang-Huo and Turmeric Formula	Jian Pi Tang
43	Rehmannia and Dogwood Fruit Formula	Ming Mu Di Huang Wan
44	Rehmannia and Magnetitum Formula	Er Ming Zuo Ci Wan
45	Rehmannia Eight	Ba Wei Di Huang Wan
46	Rehmannia Six	Liu Wei Di Huang Wan
47	Rhubarb and Scutellaria Formula	Li Dan Pian
48	Stephania and Astragalus Formula	Fang Ji Huang Qi Tang
49	Tang Gui and Gardenia Formula	Wen Qing Yin
50	Tang Gui and Ginseng Eight	Ba Zhen Tang
51	Tang Gui and Indigo Formula	Chien Chin Chih Tai Wan
52	Tang Gui Four	Si Wu Tang
53	Tian Qi and Eucommia Formula	Tin Tzat To Chung Pills
54	Tu-Huo and Loranthus Formula	Du Huo Ji Sheng Tang
55	Xanthium and Magnolia Formula	Bi Yan Pian

Index

About the Author

David Molony is currently the executive director of the American Association of Oriental Medicine and served on its board of directors from 1992 to 1996. He received a diploma in Traditional Chinese Medicine from the San Francisco College of Acupuncture and Oriental Medicine. In addition, he has completed advanced studies in Western Herbology (*The California School for Herbal Studies*, Forestville, CA), acupuncture (*Nanjing College of Traditional Chinese Medicine*, People's Republic of China), and homeopathy (*The Atlantic Academy of Homeopathy*, New York City) and has done clinical rotations with herbs at the Traditional Chinese Medicine hospital in Nanjing. In 1992, Dr. Molony received a Ph.D. in Oriental Medicine from the College of Medicina Alternativa in Columbo, Sri Lanka. He is currently enrolled in a three-year Acupuncture Orthopedics program. He and his wife, Dr. Ming Ming Pan Molony, have a private practice in Catasauqua, Pennsylvania.